Advanced Practice Nurses

The Jones and Bartlett Series in Nursing

Advanced Practice Nurses

Education, Roles, Trends

Ada Romaine-Davis, PhD, RN, CANP

Johns Hopkins University School of Nursing
Baltimore, Maryland

Jones and Bartlett Publishers
Sudbury, Massachusetts
Boston   London   Singapore

Editorial, Sales, and Customer Service Offices

Jones and Bartlett Publishers
40 Tall Pine Drive
Sudbury, MA 01776
508-443-5000
info@jbpub.com
http://www.jbpub.com

Jones and Bartlett Publishers International
Barb House, Barb Mews
London W6 7PA
UK

Library of Congress Cataloging-in-Publication Data

Romaine-Davis, Ada, 1929–
     Advanced practice nurses : education, roles, trends / Ada Romaine-Davis
     p.   cm.
     Includes bibliographical references and index.
     ISBN 0-07-637037-2
     1. Nursing specialties—United States.   2. Nurse practitioners—
United States.   I. Title.
     [DNLM: 1. Nurse Practitioners—education—United States.   2. Nurse
Clinicians—education—United States.   3. Nurse Midwives—education—
United States.   4. Nurse Anesthetists—education—United States.
     5. Specialties, Nursing—trends—United States.   WY 18 R757a 1997]
     RT86.73.R66   1997
     610.73'6—dc21
     DNLM/DNC
     for Library of Congress   97-1397
                                                                                            CIP

Production Editor: Marilyn E. Rash
Manufacturing Manager: Dana L. Cerrito
Production Service: BookMasters, Inc.
Typesetting: BookMasters, Inc.
Cover Design: Hannus Design Associates
Cover Printing: Coral Graphic Services, Inc.
Printing and Binding: Edwards Brothers

Printed in the United States of America
01   00   99   98   97   10   9   8   7   6   5   4   3   2   1

Contents

Preface

The intended readers of this book include all those interested in finding out about nurses who comprise the group now known as Advanced Practice Nurses (APNs). These readers may be prospective nursing students and their families, physicians and other health professionals who want specific information about APNs, and nursing students just being introduced to the profession of nursing.

The purpose of this book is to describe and differentiate the four components which, today, comprise the concept of *advanced practice nursing*. The American Nurses' Association (ANA) had defined the APN as one who has additional education and skills and greater specialization than other registered nurses. The four components of advanced practice nursing are: (1) nurse practitioners (NPs), (2) certified nurse-midwives (CNMs), (3) clinical nurse specialists (CNSs), and (4) certified registered nurse anesthetists (CRNAs).

Each component has unique qualifications, knowledge, and skills, and nurses in the four areas practice within relatively well-defined boundaries. Specialties developed on the basis of documented health-care needs of particular groups of people. Current and emerging health-care needs remain the major force behind the development and continuation of these and other nursing specialties.

In the chapters that follow, each component of advanced practice nursing is examined and described in detail regarding admission requirements to the various programs for interested prospective students; the many types of NP specialty programs available; specific information, including curriculums, about the programs; delineation of the functions and skills of graduates of all programs; barriers to practice; a discussion of current issues regarding reimbursement and legal and ethical issues; professional expectations for each specialty; the professional organizations and journals associated with each specialty area, and the trends that are likely to have great impact on health care and nursing care during the next century.

The author is a licensed RN and NP who lives and practices in Maryland. Throughout this book she uses (with permission from the publications' agencies) Maryland nursing codes, regulations, and procedures as examples, not as models.

Part I

Overview

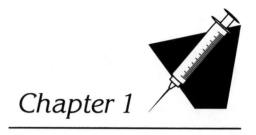

Chapter 1

Aspects of Nursing Common to All Nurses

History
Education
Professional Organizations
ANA Code of Ethics

HISTORY

The professions derived from the university traditions and from the guilds and professional groups of the Middle Ages. The original meaning of "to profess" was to take the vows of a religious order—"to be professed." In the course of time, its meaning became "the process of becoming qualified." Although initially linked to religious orders, the professions became formally associated with universities, such as the University of Paris, the University of Bologna, and others that were emerging in the very early Middle Ages. The traditional university areas of study were law, theology, and medicine. From about the tenth to the nineteenth century, persons wishing to study one of these disciplines were placed, or chose to be placed, in an apprenticeship with an acknowledged expert in the field. For example, a well-known and highly respected midwife in sixteenth-century Paris, Louise Bourgeois (1563–1653), was mentored by the famous surgeon, Ambroise Paré. In Williamsburg, Virginia, during the time preceding and following the Revolutionary War, young men who wished to study law enrolled in the College of William and Mary with the hope of reading law with notable lawyers such as George Whythe and William Randolph.

The health-care professions, however, remained somewhat outside the traditional academic community. The nursing profession, particularly, is often considered not a legitimate academic field of study. The major differences between the academic world and the health-care professions is the need for health-care providers to devote most of their academic study time in developing clinical judgment and skills, not in developing basic research knowledge and skills—the central core of traditional academic study. Thus, nursing, for many centuries, was in the lowest ranks of professional occupations; its early status continues even today, despite outstanding accomplishments of nurses in the academic setting, including scholarly, sound research in psychosocial and clinical fields of study. Nursing has struggled against occupational and gender bias to establish itself as a profession. Ironically, the increasing numbers of men entering the nursing profession may be the major factor in eliminating both occupational and gender bias in the decades ahead.

To be considered professionals, members of a group must meet the criteria defining professional status:

1. The professional is engaged in a full-time occupation that comprises his or her principal source of income. Professionals have a strong motivation ("calling") to the occupation manifested by a lifetime commitment.

2. The professional possesses a specialized body of knowledge and skills acquired during a prolonged period of formal education and training.

3. The professional makes decisions on behalf of a client by means of a clearly defined, yet broad foundation of theoretic knowledge and expertise in clinical application of knowledge and skills.

4. The professional has a service orientation, which implies diagnostic skills, competent application of general knowledge to the special needs of the client, and an absence of self-interest or self-promotion.

5. The professional's service to the client is assumed to be based on the objective needs of the client and independent of the particular sentiments that the professional may have about the client. The professional arrives at a "detached" diagnosis and is expected to withhold moral judgment about the client's revelations and diagnosis.

6. The professional demands autonomy in actions and judgment. He or she subscribes to standards judged by a panel of peers. Legal protection is sought through political influence.

7. Professional associations define criteria for admission, educational standards, licensing, entry examinations, and areas of jurisdiction for the profession. Ultimately, the professional association's function is to protect the autonomy of the profession by developing reasonable, strong forms of self-government and by establishing rules and standards for the profession.

EDUCATION

Basic nursing education forms the core of preparation for all advanced practice nurses. In the past, the basic nursing education program was that offered in three-year, hospital-based diploma schools of nursing, which was the predominant form of nursing education from the late 1880s until the early 1950s. Today, the number of three-year diploma programs has decreased to such an extent that their requirements and curriculums are not addressed here.

In 1950, during the post-World War II period of rapidly developing community colleges, Mildred Montag, a doctoral student at Columbia University, proposed in her dissertation that the education of technical nurses could take place within two-year associate degree programs. The nursing profession had worked diligently for over 50 years to establish itself as an academic program within colleges and universities, without success. Dr. Montag believed that developing nursing programs in community colleges would open the doors of the nation's four-year colleges and universities. Nursing leaders regularly, every 20 years, proclaimed that the Bachelor of Science (BS) degree should be the entry-level education for professional nurses. That dream is still to be realized, although the majority of professional nurses today recognize that without the BS degree, advancement in the nursing field is virtually impossible. However, nursing education provides a "ladder" approach. Individuals may earn, first, an Associate in Science degree (AS) in nursing, which requires completion of at least 60 academic credits. They may then apply to a college or university that offers the Bachelor of Science in Nursing (BSN) program and earn an additional 60 to 65 credits at the junior- and senior-year (upper division) level to achieve the baccalaureate degree.

Both associate- and baccalaureate-degree programs provide the theoretical and clinical components required to prepare graduates to take the state board of nursing licensing examination, known as the National Council Licensing Examination (NCLEX), to become registered nurses (RNs) within the state in which they take the examination. RNs are prepared to practice as generalists; that is, their educational program has provided both theory and practice in all areas of traditional nursing: medicine, surgery, pediatrics, obstetrics, psychiatry, and public health.

The reader should keep in mind three things regarding the discussions of schools of nursing curriculums presented in this book: (1) *examples* of curriculums, based on existing programs, are presented; programs vary with respect to didactic and clinical requirements; (2) nursing curriculums are continually changing to adjust to advances in the sciences and in medicine, surgery, and technology; and (3) at this time, admission to all nursing programs—associate degree, baccalaureate degree, and master's degree—is highly competitive.

Associate Degree Programs

Admission Requirements

To satisfy minimum qualifications for admission, candidates need to show evidence of no tubercular disease by test or chest x-ray, show evidence of booster vaccination for measles/mumps/rubella, and vaccination for hepatitis B. The specific admission requirements are:

1. Submit a completed application.
2. Meet *one* of the following requirements for secondary education:
   a. Be a graduate of a secondary school or show satisfactory completion of the General Equivalency Diploma (GED) examination.
   b. Be 18 years of age or older.
   c. Be a secondary school student who has completed the junior year with an overall 2.75 quality point average based on a 4.0 scale (Early Placement).
   d. Be a secondary school student who does not meet the requirements of the Early Placement program, but whose achievement in a certain field of study is clearly exceptional and surpasses the courses offered by the school attended and neighboring schools with alternative course choices. The college may admit such students on the recommendation of the high school counselor and the principal.
   e. Have been a student in attendance at another college or university during the semester prior to admission to the college.

Course Requirements

Human Anatomy and Physiology I (4 cr)
Chemistry for the Health Sciences (4 cr)
Fundamentals of Nursing (7 cr)
Nursing Perspectives I (3 cr)
General Psychology (3 cr)
Human Anatomy and Physiology II (4 cr)
Techniques of Reading and Writing (3 cr)
Nursing in Major Health Problems I, A and B (8 cr)*
Human Growth and Development During the Life Span (3 cr)
Microbiology (4 cr)
Techniques of Reading and Writing or Technical Writing (3 cr)
Nursing in Major Health Problems II (9 cr)*
Nursing Perspectives II (1 cr)

---

*Asterisk designates course has both didactic and clinical components.

Nursing in Major Health Problems III (10 cr)*
Introduction to Sociology (3 cr)
Humanities Distribution (3 cr)
Total credits: 70

Bachelor of Science Degree Programs

In 1992, about 671,399 (30%) of all RNs (2,239,816) had bachelor's degrees.[1]
Most BSN programs are situated in schools of nursing that offer upper division (junior and senior years) courses leading to a BSN degree. Students have the choice of taking the freshman and sophomore year requirements at a community college or in the college or university offering the BSN degree.

Admission Requirements
1. Completion and submission of application.
2. Official college transcripts of previous coursework (60 credits).
3. GPA of at least 3.0 on a 4.0 scale. (Some schools stipulate 2.75.)
4. Letters of recommendation from three persons, two of which must be from instructors in current or recent courses.
5. Official secondary school transcript (high school) unless applicant has already earned a college degree.
6. Test scores from the Scholastic Aptitude Tests (SAT) or the American College Testing Program (ACT), taken not more than five years previously.
7. A personal interview with school of nursing faculty, arranged by appointment. (Not a requirement in all schools.)

Curriculum
Courses required in the freshman and sophomore years (curriculum adjustments are made for RNs and applicants taking a second degree):

Humanities (9 cr)
English Composition (3 cr)
American or English Literature (3 cr)
Logic, Philosophy, or Ethics (3 cr) (may also be in foreign language, mathematics, history of art, or music)
Social Science (15 cr)
Psychology (3 cr)
Sociology (3 cr)
Human Growth and Development (3 cr)

---

*Asterisk designates course has both didactic and clinical components.

Anthropology, history, family or community sociology, geography, economics, political science, psychology (6 cr total)
Natural Sciences
Chemistry with laboratory component (inorganic and organic chemistry preferred) (6–8 cr)
Human Anatomy and Physiology (6–8 cr)
Microbiology (3–4 cr)
Nutrition (3 cr)
Electives (15–18 cr)
Statistics (3 cr) (generally required)
Music, studio arts, physical education (only one is transferable)

Courses required in the junior and senior (upper division) level:

Dimensions of the Nursing Role (4 cr)*
Nursing in the Health Care System (3 cr)
Principles and Applications I, II (2 cr each)*
Computers in Nursing (2 cr)
Pathophysiology (3 cr)
Pharmacology (2 cr)
Nursing: Maternal-Child (4 cr)*
Nursing: Pediatrics (4 cr)*
Research Process (3 cr)
Biostatistics (3 cr)
Nursing: Adults (4 cr)*
Psychopathology (3 cr)
Nursing: Adult Emotional Health (3 cr)*
Nursing: Community Health (4 cr)*
Leadership: Contemporary Nursing Practice (4 cr)*
Electives (9 cr)
Total credits: 63

Master's Degree Programs

In 1992, about 168,000 (7.5%) of all RNs (2,239,816) held master's degrees.[1] The undergraduate BS degree prepares students to be generalists, that is, to practice in all areas of nursing. The master's degree program prepares the baccalaureate-prepared RN to become a specialist in some area of nursing (e.g., advanced practice nursing—nurse practitioner, nurse-midwife, clinical nurse specialist, or nurse anesthetist, acute care, cardiac care, medicine,

---

*Asterisk indicates course has both didactic and clinical components.

surgery, psychiatric nursing, pediatrics, maternal-child health, oncology, HIV/AIDS, or other specialty). Clinical nurse specialists usually receive their education in one of the master's degree specialty areas.

In general, to earn the master's degree, students are required to take a minimum of 35 credits of coursework and clinical practice. Nurse practitioners (NP), nurse-midwives (NM), and certified registered nurse anesthetists (CRNA) are required to take 45 to 60 semester credit hours; nurse anesthetist programs require the highest number of credits. NP students must have a minimum of 525 hours[2] of clinical experience under the supervision of a preceptor (NP or physician). Family NP (FNP) students are required to have a minimum of 600 hours[2] of clinical experience.

Admission Requirements
1. Completion and submission of application.
2. A BS degree in nursing from a program accredited by the National League for Nursing.
3. A GPA of 3.0 on a 4.0 scale.
4. Three letters of recommendation, two of which must be from faculty.
5. Licensure as an RN in at least one state.
6. Personal interview, by telephone or in person, by appointment.
7. At least one year of full-time clinical practice as a professional nurse (some schools/programs require two years in a specialty area, e.g., labor and delivery room, or critical/intensive care).

Curriculum
A typical program of study for a master's degree requires:

Core courses
    Concepts and Theories in Nursing (3 cr)
    Ethics of Health Care (3 cr)
    Computer Applications in Nursing (2 cr)
    Professional Issues (1 cr)
    Advanced Biostatistics (2 cr)
    Advanced Pathophysiology (3 cr)
    Research Design Methodology (3 cr)
    Thesis or Scholarly Project (4–6 cr)
Courses in major
    Acute Care (or other specialty) (12 cr)*
    Elective (3 cr)
Total credits: 36–38

---

*Asterisk indicates course has both didactic and clinical components.

Examples of curriculums for each APN specialty are included in each specialty's chapter.

In 1992, about 11,300 (0.5%) of all RNs (2,239,816) held doctoral degrees.[1] In general, doctoral programs focus on research, administration, health policy, or clinical practice.

PROFESSIONAL ORGANIZATIONS

Early in this century, nursing leaders, notably Isabel Hampton and Mary Adelaide Nutting (the first and second, respectively, directors of nursing at Johns Hopkins Hospital Training School for Nurses and Johns Hopkins Hospital), were major forces in the development of the two professional groups that have remained dominant in nursing ever since: the American Nurses' Association (ANA), and the National League for Nursing (NLN). The ANA was developed to meet the needs and set the standards of practice for the practicing nurse; the NLN was formed to oversee the accreditation of nursing schools and set standards for educational programs and curriculums. The professional organizations have been instrumental in maintaining the quality of practice and educational preparation at all levels: initially, the hospital diploma programs, then the associate, baccalaureate, and master's degree programs that have developed over the ensuing years. NLN accreditation and a state's board of nursing approval, are generally required for all nursing education programs. Professional organizations relevant to each APN specialty are described in each specialty's chapter.

ANA CODE OF ETHICS

The ANA developed a code for nurses as a guide for ethical standards of practice for nurses.[3] The code states:

1. The nurse provides services with respect for the dignity of the person, unrestricted by considerations of nationality, race, creed, color, or status.
2. The nurse safeguards the individual's right to privacy by judiciously protecting information of a confidential nature, sharing only that information relevant to the person's care.
3. The nurse maintains individual competence in nursing practice, recognizing and accepting responsibility for individual actions and judgments.
4. The nurse acts to safeguard patients when their care and safety are affected by incompetent, unethical, or illegal conduct of any person.

5. The nurse uses individual competence as a criterion in accepting delegated responsibilities and in assigning nursing activities to others.
6. The nurse participates in research activities when assured that the rights of individual subjects are protected.
7. The nurse participates in the efforts of the profession to define and upgrade standards of nursing practice and education.
8. The nurse, acting through the professional organizations, participates in establishing and maintaining conditions of employment conducive to high-quality nursing care.
9. The nurse works with members of health professions and other citizens in promoting efforts to meet health needs of the public.
10. The nurse refuses to give or imply endorsement to advertising, promotion, or sales of commercial products, services, or enterprises.

In addition, each APN specialty has developed its own code of ethics and standards for professional practice, and each has its own professional organization and journal. This information is included in each specialty's chapter.

REFERENCES

1. *1992: National Sample Survey of Registered Nurses.* Rockville, MD: Division of Nursing, Bureau of Health Professions, Health Resources and Services Administration, Public Health Service, Department of Health and Human Services, 1992. (This data changes every year.)
2. National Organization of Nurse Practitioner Faculties. *Curriculum Guidelines and Program Standards for Nurse Practitioner Education,* 2nd ed. Washington, DC: National Organization of Nurse Practitioner Faculties, 1995. (Clinical hours requirements are increasing in all programs as a result of this publication.)
3. American Nurses' Association. *American Nurses' Association Code.* Washington, DC: American Nurses' Association, 1985.

BIBLIOGRAPHY

History of Nursing

Nutting, MA. *A History of Nursing.* New York: Putnam, 1935.
Reverby, SM. *Ordered to Care: The Dilemma of American Nursing, 1850–1945.* Cambridge: Cambridge University Press, 1987.

Shryock, R. *The History of Nursing*. Philadelphia: Saunders, 1959.
Stewart, I. *A History of Nursing from Ancient to Modern Times*. New York: Putnam, 1962.
Varney, H. *Nurse-Midwifery*, 3rd ed. Boston: Blackwell Scientific, 1996.

Curriculums

The information for associate, baccalaureate, and master's degrees is based on existing curriculums from several different two-year and four-year colleges and universities. Because the curriculums are examples/composites of several, the institutions should remain anonymous.

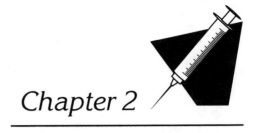

Chapter 2

Ethical Issues in Nursing

Value Systems
Ethical Systems
Clinical Research
Nurse Responsibilities

Students and graduates of education programs in the health professions are required to be knowledgeable about ethics and how to handle ethical dilemmas that inevitably arise in delivery of care. The general principles of ethics are part of all curriculums. Case studies of ethical dilemmas in the clinical area are discussed, analyzed, and are an integral part of all nursing education programs. Clinical situations may have both legal and ethical dimensions; students learn to differentiate these dimensions and address them separately.

VALUE SYSTEMS

A value is a personal belief about worth, and it acts as a standard to guide behavior. A value system is a systematic, organized pattern of values in which each value is ranked along a continuum regarding its importance relative to all other values. An individual's value system often operates as a personal code of conduct.

Generally, six types of values are recognized: (1) theoretical—the theoretical person values truth and tends to be empirical, critical, and rational; (2) economic—the economic person is interested in what is practical and useful; (3) aesthetic—the aesthetic person values beauty, form, and harmony; (4) social—the social person values people in terms of love, and is kind, sympathetic, empathetic, and unselfish (altruistic); (5) political—

the political person values power; (6) religious—the religious person values unity, ideals, philosophy, faith.

Values develop in many ways:

1. *Modeling*—children and others pattern their behavior on parents' and other persons' beliefs and values regarding what has high or low value; modeling can result in either acceptable or unacceptable behavior, depending on what is learned from the role model.

2. *Moralizing*—a method of teaching children a complete value system; the teacher can be parents, church, and/or school. In this method, the learner has little opportunity to weigh the importance of values taught; the learner is told what to do and what to believe.

3. *Laissez-faire*—children learn values on their own, with little or no teaching. Without guidance, this method often leads to confusion because of conflicting inputs, for example, when parents' behavior/values differ from the child's peers' behavior and values; the child is left wondering which is "right."

4. *Rewarding/punishing*—parents reward or punish behavior, depending on whether behavior is acceptable or unacceptable. In some cases, rewards and punishments are not explained, and children do not know why they are being rewarded or punished. When parents reward or punish arbitrarily, without giving clear reasons, children are confused and angry.

5. *Responsible choice*—children are encouraged to question and to explore different values and to see or predict their consequences. With guidance, children develop their own personal value system.

6. *Genetically determined*—recent research shows that a person's values and concept of "good" and "right" behavior and attitudes are, in part, inherited. For example, in a chaotic family in which there is no discernible value system and no guidance for children, one or more of the children grows up to have a complex, rational, acceptable value system.

In 1985, the American Association of Colleges of Nursing (AACN) concluded that seven values are essential to the practice of nursing: (1) aesthetics, (2) altruism, (3) equality, (4) freedom, (5) human dignity, (6) nonjudgment, and (7) justice.

"Value neutral" is also a desirable trait for health professionals to have. The value of neutrality is demonstrated by being "nonjudgmental."

In this way, the nurse can accept each individual, regardless of his or her values, beliefs, creeds, attitudes, and behavior. In being nonjudgmental, the health professional recognizes that all behavior occurs for a reason. Although we may not know or understand the reason behind a person's behavior, we can accept that something has caused the behavior. The nurse's task is to accept the behavior as it occurs.

Values clarification is a process by which people come to understand their own values and value system. The process involves understanding oneself and is one of exploration and discovery. This process should be an intrinsic part of every child's development, so that each one comes to know that values form the basis of who a person is and what the person stands for. Values theorists describe the process as having seven parts, divided among three activities. When one values something, one:

- chooses—(a) freely, (b) from alternatives, and (c) after careful consideration of the consequences of each alternative;
- prizes—(a) with pride and happiness, (b) with public affirmation;
- acts—(a) with incorporation of the choice into one's behavior, (b) with consistency and regularity regarding the value.

Attitudes and beliefs also influence behavior and need to be viewed as separate and distinct from values. An attitude is a feeling or an emotion, usually including positive and negative judgments, about persons, things, and/or ideas. A belief is a particular area of intellectual attitudes based largely on faith rather than on facts.

People from different cultures bring their own values, beliefs, and attitudes toward health, health care, health-care personnel, and how they wish to be treated. Health professionals need to know the cultures of many people, and to respect and respond appropriately to cultural attitudes and beliefs that are different from one's own.

ETHICAL SYSTEMS

Ethics is a systematic inquiry into the principles of right and wrong, virtue and vice, good and evil, as these relate to behavior. The Hippocratic Oath and the Nightingale Pledge are examples of codes of ethics, or proper and expected behavior. Florence Nightingale said, "First, do no harm [to the patient]."[1]

Morals, although similar to ethics, usually represent a more personal code of behavior, often based on one's religious teaching and beliefs. Often, one finds it difficult to distinguish among legal, traditional, customary, religious, and personal ethics or morals. A law may indicate what the ethical procedure(s) may be, but individuals may consider the law as not morally acceptable or right. It is equally important for persons to recognize that behaviors of others may, in their view, not be moral, but the behaviors may be within the law. The Biblical maxim, "An eye for an eye and a tooth for a tooth" connotes revenge for wrongs, but carrying out this maxim in today's world may be illegal according to our current laws. Citizens are not supposed to take the law into their own hands and mete out justice according to their own wishes.

Health professionals are often involved in ethical dilemmas—patients refusing treatment; providing care to patients with poor prognoses, often termed "futile care"; resuscitation or discontinuation of lifesaving treatment; issues around informed consent; determination of whether patients are competent to make decisions; issues about withholding information from patients; and allocation of scarce resources.

Many health-care facilities and organizations, to better resolve ethical dilemmas, have formed ethics committees—groups made up of physicians, nurses, administrators, lawyers, psychiatrists, and priests, rabbis or ministers. In special cases, additional people with expert knowledge or experience, including family members, may be brought into the group. These individuals discuss specific ethical problems brought to their attention, involving decisions about particular patients or clinical situations. Many of the problems are concerned with life-and-death outcomes, such as whether to continue treatment for terminally ill patients, whether to perform surgery in particular instances, as in the case of conjoined twins, and other situations that are especially difficult to decide on actions. Ethics committees therefore share their collective wisdom and experience in arriving at decisions. Ethical decisions are rarely "either/or" decisions; most are shrouded in doubt and uncertainty because of the complex circumstances in which they occur. There is seldom an absolute right or wrong decision; however, committees make the best decisions possible, given the circumstances of the situation, and bear the burden of the decision.

Professional codes of ethics generally include such principles as respect for persons, autonomy (self-determination), beneficence (doing good), maleficence (doing harm), veracity (telling the truth), confidentiality (respecting privileged information), fidelity (keeping promises), and justice (treating people fairly).

Although legal violations may result in legal or criminal liability for health professionals, violation of the professional code of ethics may result in reprimand, censure, suspension, or expulsion from the profession by the respective peer group as represented by a state's board of nursing.

Many situations arise about which one does not know the answer or what should be done. If professionals have doubts about what they should do in a particular situation or how they should behave, they should seek advice from their superior—the person to whom they are responsible. No matter how trivial the question seems to be, it is better to seek advice before responding. On the other hand, one's own common sense and professional competence is likely to guide the individual to the right decision most of the time.

CLINICAL RESEARCH

All nursing faculty, and many practicing nurses, engage in research, much of which is clinical research, not basic ("bench") research, the term for research conducted in biochemical laboratories. In performing clinical research, all health professionals must follow assiduously the ethical rules and regulations that are in place in the particular institution. APN faculty in universities are also required to participate in research to achieve promotion. Research studies conducted by nurses can be found in such journals as *Nursing Research, Image,* and *Research in Nursing and Health.*

The research application process to obtain government or private funds to support the research is lengthy. Part of the process involves submitting information about the research study to the Institutional Review Board (IRB), or its equivalent, such as the Joint Committee on Clinical Investigation (JCCI), which ensures that appropriate informed consent forms are in place, and that no harm to patients occurs. Approval by an IRB is required before funding is provided by the funding source. A hypothetical consent form for clinical research is shown in Exhibit 3–1.

Consent forms are required for each procedure proposed and ordered by physicians, throughout the entire period of the patient's hospitalization.

The primary focus is that the patient's autonomy (right to refuse) is safeguarded, at whatever stage of his/her illness or treatment. Such autonomy is guaranteed under the Patient's Bill of Rights, which every institution follows.

These processes have resulted from practices in the past, when patients' rights and autonomy were not always considered, for example, when groups of people were vaccinated, they neither signed a consent form, knew what they were being injected with, or the purpose of the injections.

NURSE RESPONSIBILITIES

Every practicing nurse must know the ethical standards under which a particular organization or institution operates, know the types of consent forms used under what circumstances, know the appropriate procedures for witnessing documents, and know who is responsible for obtaining con-

EXHIBIT 3–1
Example of a Consent Form

Urban Hospital
Joint Committee on Clinical Investigation

By signing this form, you state that you are willing to participate in the research project described above. If you agree to participate, you will be assigned to one of two or more groups, only one of which will be placed on the experimental drug. It is possible that the group to which you are assigned will be given a placebo, an agent that has no effect in treating the disease. Your doctors, or the investigators, explained the other kinds of treatment that are available to you and others. You should ask the principal investigator any questions you may have about this research study. You are free to ask questions at any time during the study, if you do not understand something that is being done. The investigators or your doctors will share with you any new findings that may develop while you are participating in the study.

The records from this research study will be kept confidential and will not be given to anyone who is not helping in this study, unless you agree to have the records given to others. If the study uses a new drug or device that is under the jurisdiction of the U.S. Food and Drug Administration (FDA) of the federal government, the FDA officials may look at the relevant part of your medical records as part of their responsibility to review new drug and device studies.

If you wish to talk with anyone about this research study because you think you have not been treated fairly, or think you have been hurt by joining the study, or you have any other questions about the study, you should call the principal investigator, [name] at [telephone number], or call the Office of the Joint Committee on Clinical Investigation at [telephone number]. Either the investigator or the people in the Committee office or IRB office will answer your questions and/or help you to find medical care for an injury that you feel you have suffered. This institution and the federal government do not have any program to provide compensation to you if you experience injury or other bad effects which are not the fault of the investigators.

You may withdraw from the research study at any time. Even if you do not want to join the study, or if you withdraw from it, you will still receive the same quality of medical care available to you at Urban Hospital.

If you agree to join this study, please sign your name below.

Signatures required: Subject or Parent or Guardian of the Subject, Witness to the Consent Procedure, and Investigator or Approved Designee, with date. Signed copies of the consent form are retained on file by the principal investigator, placed in the patient's medical records, and given to the patient (subject).

sent signatures of patients, particularly if the patient is confused or se-
dated. This knowledge is necessary for a nurse to protect the patient,
protect herself or himself, and protect other personnel with whom the
nurse works.

REFERENCE

1. Nightingale F. *Notes on Nursing: What It Is and What It Is Not.* London: Harrison,
   1859; New York: D. Appleton, 1960. (Reprinted, New York: Dover, 1969.)

BIBLIOGRAPHY

American College of Physicians Ethics Manual, 3rd ed. *Ann Intern Med,* 117(1):
   947–960, 1992.
American Nurses' Association. *American Nurses' Association Code.* Washington, DC:
   American Nurses' Association, 1985.
Hall, JK. *Nursing Ethics and Law.* Philadelphia: Saunders, 1996.

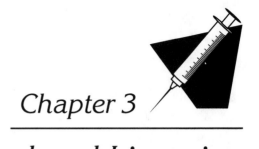

Chapter 3

Legal and Licensing Aspects of Nursing

Nurses' changing roles, responsibilities, and accountability in today's world make it essential for them to be informed about the legal and licensing implications of practice. The legal aspects of nursing are multiple and complex. Every practicing nurse should know about how the legal aspects affect one individually, and what can be done to prevent being caught in a legal net through ignorance of the law. The state's nurse practice act should be requested each year, since changes occur continuously.

The general terms and principles of the law are included as a requirement in all nursing curriculums. Practicing nurses periodically update their knowledge about current law regarding professional practice and liability. Students analyze case studies of clinical situations involving actual or potential legal implications. A *law* is a standard or rule of conduct established and enforced by the government of a society. Laws are intended chiefly to protect the rights and safety of the public. A *public law* is a law in which the government is directly involved. It regulates the relationships between individuals and the government. An important body of public law describes the powers of the government in authority. A *private law*, also called *civil law*, regulates the relationships among people. Civil law includes those laws relating to contracts, ownership of property, and the practice of medicine, nursing, dentistry, and pharmacy.

24

SOURCES OF LAW

Four sources of law exist at both the federal and state levels:

1. *Constitutions*—federal and state constitutions show how their governments are created and given authority; they state the principles and provisions for establishing specific laws. Although these documents contain relatively few actual laws (called *constitutional laws*), they serve as guides for legislative bodies.

2. *Statutes*—*statutory law* is enacted by a legislative body. In the United States, statutory laws must be in accord with the federal and state constitutions. Nurse Practice Acts are an example of statutory laws.

3. *Administrative law*—heads of government (presidents, prime ministers, state governors, city mayors, etc.) administer various agencies that, among other functions, are responsible for law enforcement. The agencies have the power to make administrative rules and regulations, in accord with already enacted laws, that must be enforced. Boards of nursing are administrative agencies at the state level. The rules and regulations that a state's board of nursing adopts become administrative laws. Another example is that of a municipal (city) board of health, which makes rules and regulations to protect the health of its citizens, such as quarantine.

4. *Common law*—evolves from written, court-made laws. *Common law* can therefore be termed *court-made law.* Law regarding malpractice is court-made law. Common law is based on the legal foundation known as *stare decisis,* or "let the decision stand." After a decision has been made in the courts, that law becomes the standard rule of practice in other, similar cases. The first case in which the decision was made is called a *precedent.* Law made in the court system is difficult to change unless there is very strong justification for the change. On the other hand, common law is more flexible and can be applied across cases of a similar nature. "Common law" marriages exist, for example, if a couple has been living together for a minimum of seven years, (perhaps) has children, and is thus "married" in every sense except legally. Courts of law acknowledge common-law marriages in terms of property rights or inheritance.

LITIGATION

Litigation is the process of carrying through on a lawsuit. The person or group bringing suit against another is the "plaintiff," the one with a cause or complaint against another. The one being accused of a crime or tort is the "defendant." In the United States, the defendant is presumed innocent until proven guilty of crime *alleged* to have been committed.

COURT SYSTEM

Two levels of courts exist in the United States: (1) trial court, or first-level court, and (2) appellate court. The trial court hears all the evidence in a case and makes decisions based on facts, generally by means of a jury, which is a group of objective persons.

The appellate court hears only cases questioning a point of law already decided by trial court. No witnesses testify at the appellate court level. However, the decisions of appellate court judges are published *and become common law.*

CRIMES AND TORTS

A *crime* is a wrong against a person or the property of a person, but the act is also considered to be against the public. In a criminal case, the government ("the people"), prosecutes the offender ("criminal"). When a person commits a crime, whether the person intended to commit the crime is irrelevant. The fact that the crime was committed is sufficient to make the person guilty. Ignorance of the law is not an excuse for breaking the law. In most cases, criminal law is statutory law; only rarely is it common law.

Crimes are classified as felonies or misdemeanors. A *misdemeanor* is a crime that is less serious than a felony. A *felony* is punishable by imprisonment in a state or federal penitentiary for more than one year. A *tort* is also a wrong committed by a person against another person or the property of another person. Torts usually result in civil trials. The court in a civil trial case settles damages with money but rarely by imprisonment.

Intentional Torts

Intentional torts include such actions as assault and battery, defamation of character, invasion of privacy, false imprisonment, and fraud. One committing a tort is presumed to have knowledge of the allowable legal limits of the wrong action, either words or deeds. Therefore, violating the known limits is grounds for prosecution.

Assault and battery is an example of an intentional tort. Assault is a threat or an attempt to make bodily contact with a person without that person's consent. Battery is an assault that is carried out and includes every willful, angry, and violent or negligent touching of another person's body, clothes, or anything that is held by or attached to that person (such as jewelry or a purse).

If a nurse (or anyone else) must make a defense against an assaultive patient or person, the nurse can use only the actions necessary for self-protection. Undue force or actual striking of the assaultive patient or person may be regarded as an act of battery.

Informed consent is required for any invasive diagnostic or treatment modality. On admission to a care facility, a patient must sign a consent form even to receive routine care. If specific invasive procedures must be done, a form must be signed for each test or treatment. The patient must, in addition to reading about the procedure on the consent form, receive an oral explanation about the procedure in sufficient detail for him/her to understand what is to happen, and why. The physician or person who will perform the procedure is responsible for giving the oral explanation to the patient. The nurse signs the form only as a witness to having seen the patient sign the form, not as the one responsible for obtaining the patient's signature. The consent form involves several aspects:

1. *Disclosure*—communication, that is, the patient has been told (1) about the current medical status and course of treatment; (2) about the risks and benefits of various treatment alternatives; (3) that no outcomes can be guaranteed; and (4) the professional opinion as to the best alternative for treatment.

2. *Comprehension*—understanding, that is, (1) the physician or nurse has provided appropriate information in a way that is clearly understandable to the patient, considering the patient's age, impairments (if any), level of education, and the like; (2) possible barriers to understanding (pain, anxiety, medication) have been assessed; (3) outside barriers to understanding (culture, language, speed, and clarity of presentation) have been assessed.

3. *Competence*—the nurse (1) assesses the competence of the patient to understand; (2) assesses the requirement of the task; (3) assesses the possible bad effects of the patient's decision; (4) determines that the patient possesses a set of values and goals that make it possible for him/her to make reasonably consistent choices; (5) determines that the patient is able to communicate and understand the information presented; and (6) determines that the patient has the ability to reason and deliberate.

4. *Voluntariness*—the nurse (1) determines that the patient has not been forced to consent; (2) avoids coercive influences by self or others; and (3) avoids subtle manipulation of the patient by self or others.

Failure to obtain a consent form can result in charges of battery brought by the patient or the patient's family against the hospital, physician(s), or nurse(s) involved.

Defamation of character is an intentional tort in which one party makes derogatory remarks about another, thus diminishing the other party's reputation. *Slander* is an untruthful, oral statement about a person that subjects that person to ridicule or contempt. *Libel* is written defamation.

Defamation of character is grounds for an award of civil damages, with the amount of the award based on the degree of harm done the plaintiff. Nurses who make false statements about their patients or co-workers run the risk of being sued for slander or libel. A person charged with slander or libel may not be liable if it can be proved that the statement was made not to injure another but for some nonmalicious, justifiable purpose, such as proof of consent, truth, privilege, or fair comment.

Invasion of privacy is ensured by the Fourth Amendment of the U.S. Constitution, which protects citizens by giving them the right of privacy and the right to be left alone. Disclosure of confidential information whenever a patient's problem is inappropriately discussed with a third party may be construed as *invasion of privacy*. The nurse's intimate knowledge of the patient and his/her condition places the nurse at greater risk in this regard. Invasion of privacy should be claimed in instances such as (1) unnecessary exposure of the patient during transfer or in providing physical care; (2) talking with patients in rooms that are not soundproof; (3) discussing information about the patient to persons not entitled to such information (e.g., other patients, any professional not officially part of the patient's care, the press, etc.); and (4) carrying out research without taking proper precautions to ensure patients' anonymity.

False imprisonment is unjustified retention or prevention of movement of another person without proper consent. Using reasonable methods of restraint when absolutely needed, retaining a patient in a hospital or other facility without that person's consent when the person is not harmful to him/herself or to others, can all be grounds for charges of false imprisonment.

Fraud is willful and purposeful misrepresentation that could cause, or has caused, loss or harm to a person or property. Misrepresentation of a product is a common fraudulent act. Misrepresenting the possible outcome of treatment or procedure may constitute fraud.

Unintentional Torts

Negligence and Malpractice
Negligence is defined as performing an act that a reasonably prudent person under similar circumstances would not do or, conversely, failing to perform an act that a reasonably prudent person under similar circum-

stances would do. Therefore, negligence comprises acts of omission and commission.

Malpractice is the term used to describe negligence by professional personnel.

Elements of liability consist of four components that must be established to prove that malpractice or negligence occurred: (1) *duty*—an obligation to use due care (what a reasonably prudent person would do) as defined by the standard of care appropriate for the nurse-patient relationship; (2) *breach of duty*—the failure to meet the standard of care; (3) *causation*—the action that is the failure to meet the standard of care (breach) or the action that causes injury (the component that is the most difficult to prove); and (4) *damages*—the actual harm or injury to the patient resulting from the action.

Standards of care are based on actions that a reasonably prudent nurse would do under similar circumstances.

Malpractice Litigation

When a patient or other person pursues legal action and claims that the patient was injured through the negligence of a nurse, one of three outcomes usually ensues: (1) all parties concerned work toward a fair settlement; (2) the case is presented to a malpractice arbitration panel; or (3) the case is brought to trial court.

The most frequent allegations against nurses include:

- failure to ensure patient safety
- improper treatment or performance of treatment
- failure to monitor and to report
- medication errors and reactions
- failure to follow hospital procedure
- failure to document adequately or appropriately
- improper use of equipment
- discrimination against particular groups of patients, such as HIV/ AIDS patients
- transmission of nosocomial infections
- breach of confidentiality.

Student nurses are responsible for their own acts of negligence if their actions result in patient injury. The nursing instructor and the student may share responsibility for damages in the event of patient injury if the student's assignment called for clinical skills beyond the student's competency or if the instructor failed to provide reasonable and prudent supervision. Because changes in patients' status can occur rapidly, especially in the hospital setting, a student must report any perceived changes in patients' condition, even if the student is not sure of the importance or meaning of the changes.

PROFESSIONAL AND LEGAL REGULATION OF NURSING

Both voluntary and legal controls map the boundaries of nursing practice. The controls are designed to protect society from unsafe nursing practice and to promote the highest possible quality of care.

Voluntary controls are controls that the professional organizations develop as guidelines for peer review. Examples of voluntary standards are the ANA's Standards of Nursing Practice. (The Canadian Nurses' Association has the same or similar guidelines for standards of practice.) These professional organizations provide accreditation of programs and service organizations.

Legal standards are developed by legislative action and implemented by authority granted by the state (e.g., to a board of nursing). Legal standards usually provide for the *minimal* level of practice deemed essential for the safety of patients. The bestowal of a license to individuals indicates that that person has, by means of written examination and previous educational performance, met the requirements and is qualified to provide safe care at the minimal level as stipulated by the law. The states pass laws (Nurse Practice Acts) and then issue regulations that stipulate how the laws are to be carried out. It is not sufficient to know only the practice acts; one must also know the regulations around the nurse practice acts. When one requests a copy of a state's nurse practice act, one must also request the regulations.

Credentialing

Credentialing is the means by which the profession ensures the quality and safety of care provided by nurses. The term refers to the ways in which professional competence is ensured and maintained. Three processes are involved in credentialing:

1. *Accreditation*—the process by which an educational program is evaluated and then recognized as having met certain predetermined standards of education. Accreditation of an educational program by the NLN is voluntary. However, legal accreditation of educational programs is required through state boards, such as the board of nursing, which also evaluate and accredit education programs.

2. *Licensure*—the process by which a state determines that a candidate meets certain minimal requirements to practice in the profession and then grants a license to practice. Some states grant a license to nurses who qualify as APNs.

3. *Certification*—the process by which a person who has met certain criteria established by a nongovernmental association is granted recognition. For example, a nurse with particular qualifications may take the ANCC adult nurse practitioner (NP) certification examination to be certified nationally. Individual states may require an NP to take state certification examinations to practice as an NP in that state. Most states accept the ANCC certification as sufficient qualification for practice.

LICENSURE AND REGISTRATION

A license is a legal document that permits a person to offer to the public their skills and knowledge in a particular jurisdiction in which such practice would be unlawful without a license. All states require a license to practice as a physician, nurse, pharmacist, dentist, or other type of health professional who provides hands-on care or treatment. Once the individual passes the licensing examination, the name of the individual is registered in the state's records. The person must renew the license/registration periodically (usually annually) according to the state's laws.

A license can be suspended for a period of time or revoked permanently because of drug or alcohol abuse, which renders the person unfit and unable to practice safely because of impaired cognitive and physical abilities. Other causes for suspension or revocation are fraud, deceptive practices, criminal acts, previous disciplinary action by other state boards, gross or ordinary negligence, and physical and mental impairments such as those that occur as a result of aging.

However, once earned, a license to practice is a property (ownership) right, and cannot be revoked without due process. *Due process* entails notice of the investigation, a fair and impartial hearing, and a proper decision based on substantial evidence. Critical to a nurse's successful defense are early legal counsel, use of character and expert witnesses, and thorough preparation for all proceedings.

History

State nurse practice acts were developed early in the twentieth century; North Carolina enacted the first nurse registration act in 1903. The act provided that, from 1904, only individuals who were listed with the North Carolina Board of Examiners could identify themselves as registered nurses (RNs). Twenty years later, in 1923, similar laws were in effect in all states and the District of Columbia.

State nurse practice acts were based on the American Medical Association's Texas Medical Practice Act, first passed in 1873. This law was a benchmark, since it initiated the laws by which physicians would be licensed to practice medicine. Opposition to such laws came from physicians themselves, who believed that government did not have the right to require licensure for doctors to practice their profession. However, in 1889, in the case of *Dent v. West Virginia,* in which a similar attempt to pass a state practice act was challenged, the U.S. Supreme Court upheld the constitutionality of the West Virginia Medical Practice Act, citing the Tenth Amendment to the U.S. Constitution, which states that, "The powers not delegated to the United States by the Constitution, nor prohibited by it to the States, are reserved to the States respectively, or to the people." This Amendment supports states' powers, including the right to regulate the public health, welfare, and safety of the people. Following this landmark decision, states reacted quickly to adopt compulsory licensure laws for physicians. By 1905, 39 states had enacted medical practice laws that required physicians to obtain a license before practicing medicine in a particular state.

These efforts paved the way for formal state regulation of nursing. The Bulloughs[1] identified three distinct phases in the development of nurse practice acts in this country:

1903 to 1938:   Enactment of nurse registration acts in many states.

1938 to 1971:   State legislatures begin defining the scope of nursing practice.

1971 to present: Enhanced recognition by states of expanded roles and advanced practice and registered nurse specialties (e.g., nurse anesthetists).

Currently, the ANA's Model Practice Act (8 section 201[d])[2] recognizes all nursing specialties and defines "professional nursing practice" in part, as:

> Professional nursing practice encompasses the full scope of nursing practice and includes all its specialties and consists of application of nursing theory to the development, implementation, and evaluation of plans of nursing care for individuals, families, and communities. Professional nursing practice requires substantial knowledge of nursing theory and related scientific, behavioral, and humanistic disciplines.

Recent Trends

Despite the ANA's position to have nurse practice acts grant all practitioners a broad scope of practice, but leave specific regulation of specialties to professional organizations, recent trends show that some states have increased specific regulations for nurse practitioners (NPs), nurse-midwives, and certified nurse anesthetists. Maryland's Nurse Practice Act, for example, does not include specific regulations for clinical nurse specialists, including psychiatric clinical nurse specialists, although other states may include this area of specialization in their regulations. Practicing nurses' experience has shown that if nurses rely on broad definitions of nursing practice, their scope of practice can be more easily challenged by other health professionals. States tend to defer to the professional organizations regarding certification and accreditation of educational programs.

The primary rationale for mandatory licensure laws is protection of the public's health and welfare. Many believe that mandatory licensure is the most restrictive type of state-granted credential by requiring that individuals obtain a license before they can practice in their profession. Often, the scope of practice of the specific professional is delineated, which thereby protects both the professional title (e.g., RN or MD) and the practice. Unauthorized use of the title or practicing without a license are punishable by sanctions such as reprimand, suspension of license, revocation of license, fines, or other means. Criminal sanctions may also apply, depending on the nature of the infringement.

Because of the rebuttal by many that mandatory licensure is unnecessary and unwarranted, some states now require groups seeking passage of mandatory licensure legislation to provide rationale for licensure, rather than alternative options such as registration, certification, or no regulation.

Most state nurse practice acts stipulate the scope of practice for NPs and physician assistants (PAs). Because there is such variability among the states regarding what is considered to be appropriate scope of practice, the legal restrictions on scope of practice sometimes seriously impede health professionals from practicing within their full capabilities as provided by their educational background. The Institute of Medicine (IOM) Committee, in their 1996 report,[3] recommended that state governments review current restrictions posed by the nurse practice act, to allow NPs and PAs to practice according to their preparation. The IOM report also emphasizes the need for active collaboration and cooperation among all health professionals.

COMPETENT PRACTICE

Competent practice is the nurse's most important and best legal safeguard. Each nurse is responsible for making sure that educational background and clinical experience are adequate to fulfill the nursing responsibilities described in the job description. Legal safeguards include:

1. Respecting the legal boundaries of practice
2. Following institutional procedures and policies
3. Recognizing one's personal strengths and weaknesses and seeking a means of growth through education, supervised experience, and discussions with colleagues
4. Evaluating proposed assignments and refusing to accept responsibilities for which one is unprepared
5. Keeping current with changing standards of care and responsibilities
6. Reporting adverse incidents promptly without assuming, voicing, or recording any blame for the incident.

STATE BOARD OF NURSING ACTIONS

All state nurse practice acts contain a section that indicates the possible penalties for infractions of the law. For example, Section 8-316 of the Maryland Nurse Practice Act states:[4]

Denials, reprimands, suspensions, and revocations—grounds; additional monetary penalty; surrender of suspended or revoked license; publication of notice of revocation or suspension

(a) . . . the Board may deny a license to any applicant, reprimand any licensee, place any licensee on probation, or suspend or revoke the license of a licensee if the applicant or licensee:

The following are selected examples from 28 infractions.

(1) Fraudulently or deceptively obtains or attempts to obtain a license for the applicant or for another
(2) Fraudulently or deceptively uses a license; . . .
(4) Is convicted of or pleads guilty or *nolo contendere* to a felony or to a crime involving moral turpitude, whether or not any appeal or other proceeding is pending to have the conviction or plea set aside;
(5) Willfully and knowingly:
　(i) Files a false report or record of an individual under the licensee's care
　(ii) Gives any false or misleading information about a material matter in an employment application;

    (iii) Fails to file or record any health record that is required by law;

    (iv) Obstructs the filing or recording of any health record as required by law, or

    (v) Induces another person to fail to file or record any health record as required by law; . . .

  (7) Knowingly does any act that has been determined by the Board, in its rules and regulations, to exceed the scope of practice authorized to the individual under this title; . . .

(13) Knowingly fails to report suspected child abuse in violation of Section 5–704 of the Family Law Article; . . .

(22) Delegates nursing acts or responsibilities to an individual that the applicant or licensee knows or has reason to know lacks the ability or knowledge to perform; . . .

(25) Engages in conduct that violates the professional code of ethics;

(26) Is professionally incompetent; . . .

REFERENCES

1. Bullough VL, Bullough B. *History, Trends, and Politics of Nursing.* Norwalk, CT: Appleton-Century-Crofts, 1984.
2. American Nurses' Association. *Model Practice Act.* Washington, DC: American Nurses Publishing, 1996 (revised edition).
3. Lohn KN, Vanselow NA, Detmer DE, eds. *The Nation's Physician Workforce: Options for Balancing Supply and Requirements.* Washington, DC: Institute of Medicine, National Academy Press, 1996.
4. Maryland State Board of Nursing. *Nurse Practice Act. Annotated Code of Maryland Health Occupation Article, Title 8. Code of Maryland Regulations Title 10, Subtitle 27.* Baltimore: Maryland State Board of Nursing, 1995, p. 18.

BIBLIOGRAPHY

Most of the historical content was derived from Bullough and Bullough (cited above). Additional bibliographic sources:

Hall JK. *Nursing Ethics and the Law.* Philadelphia: Saunders, 1996.

Shryock R, *The History of Nursing.* Philadelphia: Saunders, 1959.

Stewart I, *A History of Nursing from Ancient to Modern Times.* New York: Putnam, 1962.

Part II

Advanced Practice Nursing

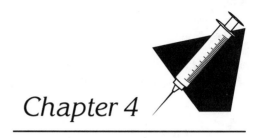

Chapter 4

Evolution of Advanced Practice Nursing

History
Definition
Areas of Responsibility
Value to Health-Care Community
Summary

In 1992, the American Nurses' Association (ANA) concluded that, for various reasons, particularly to clarify and enhance the understanding of nurses and the public about the specialized areas of nursing practice, one broad title should encompass the four advanced nursing specialties: nurse practitioner (NP), certified nurse-midwife (CNM), clinical nurse specialist (CNS), and certified registered nurse anesthetists (CRNA). According to the 1992 *National Sample Survey of Registered Nurses,* there were at that time 48,237 NPs, 7,405 CNMs, 58,185 CNSs, and 25,238 CRNAs. In all groups, about 86% of the total number were employed in nursing. The percentage nationally certified was: NPs, 58%; CNMs, 100%; CNSs, 13.5%, and CRNAs, 100%.[1]

The title selected by the ANA was Advanced Practice Nursing (APN). Areas of concern and professional issues would be addressed for all specialties, particularly when responding to political and legislative groups, as a means of showing that the specialty nursing groups were speaking "with one voice." However, because the four specialty groups did not wish to lose their individual identities, they continue to be designated by their previous names.

HISTORY

Advanced practice nursing has evolved slowly over the past three decades. Nurse anesthetists have been a professional group since the mid-

1800s and they were educated primarily by physicians and nurses who had a special interest and expertise in anesthesia in what was an apprenticeship method. Medical residencies in anesthesiology came into existence only after World War II, although many physicians were able to administer anesthesia before that time.

Mainstream nursing did not accept that CRNAs and NPs were really nurses, because they had been trained primarily by physicians and surgeons and therefore did not fit the mold of nurse. The dichotomy among persons within the profession hindered progress in the specialties and introduced a measure of divisiveness that is only now disappearing.

Recognition and acceptance of NPs came slowly. In the 1970s, schools of nursing began developing master's programs to prepare NPs. By that time, many research studies had shown the excellence and usefulness of NPs in providing care to babies and children and, later, to adults as programs expanded. Also in the early 1970s, federal funds became available to support the education of NPs, CNMs, and CNSs. A special grant program was already in place to support the education of nurse anesthetists. Nursing schools responded rapidly to federal incentives, and APN programs proliferated across the United States. At the same time, federal funding helped to promote and support primary care as a means of delivering cost-effective, comprehensive care to millions of underserved and underinsured Americans.

One of the confusing aspects of these specialties is that, although the students are now generally educated in master's programs, this was not true initially. CNSs have always been educated in master's programs, but many NPs, CNMs, and CRNAs were prepared in continuing education (CE), nondegree programs, often in schools of medicine or in the CE departments of schools of nursing. The charge made by physicians that the educational background of NPs, CNMs, and CRNAs was variable, is quite true. The situation is changing dramatically and rapidly at present, but there are still practicing APNs who do not have master's degrees. In 1992, the ANA and the American Nurses Credentialing Center (ANCC) required the master's degree for NPs applying for new or renewal certification; therefore, the number of NPs practicing without a master's degree is decreasing to zero.

DEFINITION

The ANA defined APNs in these terms:[2]

> Nurses in advanced clinical nursing practice have a graduate degree in nursing. They conduct comprehensive health assessments,

demonstrate a high level of autonomy and expert skill in the diagnosis and treatment of complex responses of individuals, families,
and communities to actual or potential health problems. Nurses in
advanced practice integrate education, research, management,
leadership, and consultation into their clinical roles and function in
collegial relationships with nursing peers, physicians, health professionals, and others who influence the health environment.

The American Academy of Nurse Practitioners also published information
and definitions similar to that issued by the ANA in 1992, stating:[3]

An advanced practice nurse has additional education and skills,
and greater specialization, than other registered nurses (RNs). Today, about 160,000 RNs have completed education beyond basic
requirements and are considered to be advanced practice nurses.

AREAS OF RESPONSIBILITY

Primary Care

Primary care was defined in the 1960s at about the time that nurses began
to be prepared as NPs, and the definition today covers a broad area of responsibility. Primary care is generally regarded as the first point of contact
of the patient with the health-care system. At that point a decision is made
about what must be done to help resolve the patient's health problem. Primary care is also continuous, comprehensive care given to all family members. Each NP has a separate caseload of families. Primary care includes all
services necessary for health promotion, prevention of disease and disability, health maintenance, and in some cases, rehabilitation. Primary
health care includes identification, management, and/or referral of people
with specific health problems that require the care of specialist physicians,
with the patient returning to the primary care provider for follow-up care
after the acute problem has been resolved. Primary care is considered
holistic care, which takes into account the needs and strengths of the individual's or family's whole system—physical, psychological, spiritual, financial, social. By its nature, primary care requires collaboration among
health professionals of all kinds and at all levels.[4]

    Primary care, therefore, bears responsibility for the vast majority—
perhaps 99%—of the health problems of the population in any given area.
Primary care is provided by family practice physicians, NPs, and others
qualified to render comprehensive, continuous care to individuals and
families. Primary care has four unique functions: (1) first-contact care, (2)
longitudinal care, (3) comprehensive care, and (4) coordination of care.

First contact means that care must be provided when it is needed. Services must be accessible in time and place and by financing and culture. Accessibility must be manifested as a behavior; the population must use the source of care in a timely manner when a need for care is perceived.

Longitudinal means that care is time-oriented rather than oriented to a disease or a disease episode. Longitudinal care is focused on a person rather than on a problem or type of problem. There must be at least an informal agreement that the patient will enroll as a regular patient and that the practitioner will be the regular source of care. Care is to be sought from the same source each time it is needed, except for specific referrals made by the primary care source to other types of providers.

Comprehensive means that there is an assumed responsibility to provide care for the most common (up to 90%) problems in the population. An explicit and appropriately inclusive range of services must be available, and the services must be provided when they are needed.

Coordination is the function that puts the pieces together when patients are referred elsewhere for procedures or therapies, with the understanding that the patient will then return to the primary care provider. The coordinating function requires some mechanisms of continuity to provide the information about care the patient receives elsewhere and requires recognition of information generated when patients must be seen in other settings for various aspects of their care. Based on the need for coordination, the role of *case manager* evolved.

The Institute of Medicine's 1996 definition of primary care is: the provision of integrated, accessible health-care services by clinicians who are accountable for addressing a large majority of personal health needs, developing a sustained partnership with patients, and practicing in the context of family and community.[5]

Other Care

APNs are a viable solution to many of the problems that exist in the health-care system. The emphasis by APNs on health promotion, disease prevention, and patient education is considered a major advantage to historical medical care, which has tended to focus on treating only specific medical conditions or illnesses.

APNs combine biological, medical, and psychosocial knowledge to treat patients holistically. Often, patients' symptoms and illness can be caused or exacerbated by psychological concerns about money, family problems, or inability to feel comfortable within the health-care system. APNs take the time to look at the whole person, to elicit information about specific worries and concerns that the patient has, which may be affecting the illness or condition that brought the patient to the clinic. Patients are made a part of the treatment process, with APNs assisting them to develop personal goals regarding weight loss, smoking, alcohol, or drug cessation. Rather than telling the patient what to do, the APN allows patients time to feel that treatment decisions are their own, not those of the provider.

APNs are skilled regarding coordination of patients' care and are generally knowledgeable about community resources and other sources of help. APNs refer patients appropriately, and follow up with the patient's treatment so that the treatment continues to be monitored and coordinated as it is needed, at the time it is needed, and that it is provided by the appropriate specialist.

VALUE TO HEALTH-CARE COMMUNITY

Because APNs tend to spend more time with patients, in some settings APNs are not considered to be as cost-effective as physicians or physician assistants, who are more problem-focused. For example, in some health maintenance organizations (HMOs), physicians and APNs are required to see patients at 15-minute intervals; many APNs have been fired for not adhering to these guidelines. Yet one cannot perform adequate histories, physical examinations, and include patient teaching about drugs and therapy within 15- or even 20-minute intervals. Health promotion and disease prevention take time. Other health-care delivery settings, however, such as physician group practices, consider these aspects of care as desirable and deliberately seek APNs to provide these aspects of care. Cross-communication between the APN and other health-care professionals can also save time for the busy specialist and for the patient.

Consumers rate the quality of care given by APNs and other specialty nurses just as highly as that received from physicians.[6] Patients also report higher satisfaction with care given by APNs in terms of personal interest, reduction of the mystique surrounding health professionals and the delivery system, the amount of information provided, and lower cost of care.[7] APNs prescribe drugs at about the same level as physicians, or lower, with higher patient satisfaction, perhaps related to the fact that APNs explain more fully the reasons for the prescription, the action of the drug, and the importance of taking the drug as prescribed.

The cost of educating APNs is much less than that required to educate physicians. The estimated cost of educating NPs in 1986 was $14,600, compared with $86,100 for educating primary care physicians in the same year. Most medical students elect to specialize in areas other than primary care (family practice). Some physicians find specialties such as cardiac surgery, rheumatology, ophthalmology, and transplant surgery more interesting and more satisfying personally and professionally than general family practice. Nurses, like family practice physicians, are more accustomed to and prefer caring for patients with multiple problems, listening to patients' complaints, and following patients over time.

Studies show that APNs can manage, at less cost, 60% to 80% of primary and preventive care traditionally done by physicians. Gerontological NPs are able to care for 80% to 95% of health problems that arise among nursing home residents, and APN care results in fewer hospitalizations and emergency room admissions, decreases use of restraints, and maximizes both physical and cognitive functioning of nursing-home residents.

Using CNMs to provide prenatal care, particularly for teenage and drug-addicted mothers, reduces overall costs of care, and results in fewer low-birth-weight babies, which lowers cost of care in neonatal intensive care units. In particular, CNMs have a lower rate of referrals for cesarean sections, which sums to a considerable cost saving for the health-care system.

APNs perform many diagnostic procedures and treatments that physicians traditionally performed, such as gynecologic examinations, throat and cervical cultures, phlebotomy, microscopic examinations of urine, sputum, and smears from various body areas. NPs who specialize in obstetrics and gynecology (Ob/Gyn) can manage the care of the majority of patients in sexually transmitted disease (STD) clinics, prenatal and postpartum clinics, and women's health clinics. The following examples show innovative and cost-effective care by APNs:[2]

> In Philadelphia, a new model for home care of very-low-birth-weight infants performed by pediatric NPs resulted in the same health outcomes as care provided in hospital neonatal intensive care units, for an average cost savings of $18,560 per infant.

> In St. Paul, MN, a "block nurse" program developed by nurses provides coordinated services to elderly people and thus allows them to remain in their homes while receiving care, at considerable cost savings.

> California has eight alternative hospitals in which APNs run the emergency room and other services; thus, only one physician is required as a consultant and to provide more complex treatment.

> In Vancouver, Washington, an NP provides health screening, immunizations, health teaching, and other services to 2000 poor children in five inner-city schools, by means of weekly visits in a mobile van equipped with x-ray, laboratory, and appropriate drugs.

In October 1994, a new clinic opened in Washington Heights-Inwood in New York City, near Columbia University. The clinic is staffed by seven NPs (four adult and three pediatric), an RN, a medical assistant, and two patient representatives who manage the clerical work. The clinic is managed by Patricia Ruiz, RN, MS, CPNP, Assistant Professor of Clinical Nursing at Columbia University School of Nursing. She also sees patients four days a week. The work entails assessment and treatment of patients of all ages, setting up programs to serve both immediate and long-range needs of areas within the nearby community, and taking advantage of all opportunities to improve the health care of the persons they serve. The clinic NPs have been awarded hospital privileges at New York's Presbyterian Hospital.

Other APN faculty throughout the United States are developing collaborative practices with physicians in primary care practices associated with schools of medicine.

SUMMARY

Changing health-care delivery systems and health-care economics, coupled with the large number of underserved, homeless, and underinsured and uninsured individuals, have coalesced to create a greater demand than ever before for the services of nurse specialists because of their high-quality, efficient, and cost-effective care.

APNs are educated to fill many roles and to collaborate with all other health professionals: physicians, social workers, therapists, administrators, and federal and state policy makers. Many of the professional organizations that have developed within the specialties work closely with local, state, and federal legislators regarding practice regulations, prescriptive privileges, legal and ethical ramifications of practice, reimbursement for services, and other issues of importance to the care and safety of the nation's people.

REFERENCES

1. *1992: National Sample Survey of Registered Nurses.* Rockville, MD: Division of Nursing, Bureau of Health Professions, Health Resources and Services Administration, Public Health Service, U.S. Department of Health and Human Services, 1992.

2. American Nurses' Association Congress of Nursing Practice, draft of publication about APNs, February 28, 1992 (rev. 1994).
3. American Academy of Nurse Practitioners, Scope of Practice for Nurse Practitioners (flyer). Washington, DC: AANP, 1992 (rev. 1993).
4. Starfield B. *Primary Care: Concept, Evaluation and Policy.* New York: Oxford University Press, 1992.
5. Institute of Medicine. *Primary Care: America's Health in a New Era.* Washington, DC: National Academy Press, 1996.
6. Letters to the Editor: Patient satisfaction. *Nurse Practitioner,* 19(6):21, 1994. *See* citations included in bibliography.
7. Letters to the Editor: Patient satisfaction. *Nurse Practitioner,* 19(6):21, 1994. *See* citations included in bibliography.

BIBLIOGRAPHY

Adamson T, Watts P. Patients' perceptions of maternity nurse practitioners. *Am J Public Health,* 66:585–586, 1976.
Batchelor G. Spitzer W, Comley A, Anderson G. Nurse practitioners in primary care: IV. Impact of an interdisciplinary team on attitudes of a rural population. *Can Med Assoc J,* 112:1415–1420, 1975.
Brown J, Brown M, Jones F. Evaluation of a nurse practitioner staffed preventive medicine program in a fee-for-service multi-specialty clinic. *Preventive Med,* 8:53–64, 1979.
Enggist R, Hatcher M. Factors influencing consumer receptivity to the nurse practitioner. *J Med Systems,* 7:495–512, 1983.
Feldman M, Ventura M, Crosby F. Studies of nurse practitioner effectiveness. *Nurs Res,* 36:303–308, 1987.
Gravely E, Littlefield J. A cost-effectiveness analysis of three staffing models for the delivery of low-risk prenatal care. *Am J Public Health,* 82:180–184, 1992.
Levine J, Orr S, Sheatsley D, Lohr J, Brodie B. The nurse practitioner: Role, physician utilization, patient acceptance. *Nurs Res,* 27:245–254, 1978.
Lewis C, Cheyovich T. Who is a nurse practitioner? Processes of care and patients' and physicians' perceptions. *Medical Care,* 14:357–364, 1976.
Linn L. Patient acceptance of the family nurse practitioner. *Medical Care,* 14: 365–373, 1976.
North N. Primary care services: In search of alternative ways of providing services that are affordable, accessible and appropriate. *Nurs Praxis N Zealand,* 6:11–18, 1991.
Office of Technology Assessment (OTA). *Nurse Practitioners, Physicians' Assistants, and Certified Nurse-Midwives: A Policy Analysis* (Health Technology Case Study No. 37). Washington, DC: U.S. Government Printing Office, 1986.
Olade R. Perception of nurses in an expanded role. *Int J Nurs Studies,* 26:15–25, 1989.

Spitzer W, Sackett D, Sibley J, et al. The Burlington randomized trial of the nurse practitioner. *N Engl J Med,* 290:153–161, 1974.

History

Kalisch PA, Kalisch BJ. *The Federal Influence and Impact on Nursing.* Hyattsville, MD: U.S. Department of Health and Human Services, Public Health Service, Health Resources Administration, Bureau of Health Professions, Division of Nursing. PHS Contract No. 1-NU-44129:446–448, 1979.

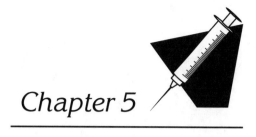

Chapter 5

Nurse Practitioner

Nurse practitioners (NPs) are registered nurses with educational preparation that is a composite of advanced nursing and primary care. The NP performs many functions traditionally performed by physicians, such as conducting physical examinations, treating acute and chronic illnesses, and providing routine care. Historically, NPs have worked outside hospitals, in community and primary care settings, and have filled the gap in areas that do not have sufficient numbers of physicians to care for the population, such as inner-city and rural areas.[1]

NP specialty areas include: adult, pediatric, family, gerontological, neonatal, community health, obstetrics and gynecology (Ob/Gyn), school, occupational health, emergency, and acute care.

HISTORY

The nurse practitioner (NP) "movement," as it is now called, began in 1965 with the development of the pediatric NP program at the University of Colorado School of Nursing's Department of Continuing Education. The program was developed collaboratively by Loretta Ford, then the dean of the school, and Henry Silver, MD, a pediatrician, both of whom recognized the need for well-baby care in Denver. Dr. Ford's vision of the NP program was "an autonomous clinical care-directed nursing model based on public health nursing principles."[2] At that time, there was a dearth of pediatricians in the region who were providing primary care. Pediatricians taught the NP students, since no qualified nurse faculty existed to teach diagnosis and management of acute and chronic illnesses of children. In addition, both Dr. Ford and Dr. Silver had the foresight to anticipate the need to evaluate the care given by the new NP graduates, and they developed a study to determine the quality and the cost-effectiveness of care by NPs.

To support the program evaluation research, Dr. Ford sought grant assistance from the federal government and subsequently received grant funds that extended over 10 years and covered three phases of the research effort. The study results showed overwhelmingly that the care given by NPs was high quality and cost effective; the study also showed that there was high satisfaction among both NPs and their patients. From this beginning, NP programs began developing rapidly in many nursing schools, spurred by the results of several other studies showing that care given by NPs was essentially equal to that given by physicians and was lower in cost.

All early NP programs were within continuing education (CE) departments, and graduates did not receive academic credit. Nursing leaders and educators were slow to accept the new role for nurses; NPs were considered "mini-docs" rather than practitioners performing the traditional roles and responsibilities of registered nurses (RNs).

However, nurses themselves saw the benefits of having additional knowledge and skills, and the number of applicants to the new programs increased rapidly. In the early to mid-1970s, schools of nursing began to develop NP programs within the academic setting and began to award academic credit. Today, almost 50,000 certified nurse practitioners in all specialties are practicing, just 31 years after the implementation of the first NP program in Colorado.

Federal funds to support NP programs became available in the 1970s. At that time, the government recognized the tremendous need for care providers in underserved areas, both inner-city and rural, and stipulated that NPs be prepared to provide care in primary care settings. The majority of RNs work in hospitals; therefore, the need for the new type of RN in hospitals was not great. Today, the knowledge and skills that NPs have are needed everywhere, largely because technological advances in medicine and surgery have escalated and because in the past two decades, hospitals have changed in character and are primarily intensive care units. In this setting, physicians and NPs are needed to make immediate, often emergency, decisions about patients' status, which tends to change rapidly and often unexpectedly. Only highly trained providers are able to assess a patient quickly and accurately and, on the basis of that assessment, decide what treatment is necessary at a particular moment. Immediate assessment and decision making allows treatment to be initiated before the patient's condition deteriorates too much for treatment to be fully effective or as effective as possible.

The change in hospitals occurred during the mid to late 1980s, when cost-containment measures were put in place by the government. The first of these measures was creation of diagnosis related groups (DRGs), which stipulated the length of stay and treatment needed for each of several hundred procedures or conditions. Patients were admitted, treated appropriately as quickly as possible, then released to recover at home. Gone were the days when patients were routinely admitted the day before surgery to undergo preoperative procedures and preparation, and when protracted periods of recovery and rehabilitation occurred before the patient was discharged. With the change in the acuity of patients' illnesses came the need for more knowledgeable and skilled care, particularly by nurses.

DEFINITION

An NP provides comprehensive, collaborative primary and specialty care for individuals, families, and communities in a variety of settings, but with special emphasis on community-based care for medically underserved populations. NPs are educated to diagnose, prescribe, and manage the total care of persons. Their area of specialization determines the range of age of patients. For example, the certified pediatric nurse practitioner (CPNP) provides total care from birth to adolescence, and the certified adult nurse practitioner (CANP) provides care to persons from adolescence to middle age and beyond, overlapping with the gerontological nurse practitioner (GNP), who cares for older persons.

In NP education, most programs of which are now master's or post-master's degree programs, adult and family NPs (FNPs) learn to diagnose and treat the spectrum of illnesses and conditions that afflict the adult population in all body systems, from high blood pressure to end-stage renal disease. Both adult and FNPs are considered to be generalists, similar to family practice physicians, although the practice of CANPs does not include care to infants and children, as does that of FNPs, except in emergency situations and according to individual capabilities as RNs. Historically, the need for CPNPs was seen in well-baby clinics in Colorado; today, NPs practice in hospitals, ambulatory care, same-day surgery, health maintenance organizations (HMOs), home health care, private practice, and other sites.

In the past five years, demand has grown for NPs in acute care (hospital) settings. Guidelines for practice, responsibility, and accountability required of NPs in these settings have been developed, and programs to prepare NPs for practice in all settings, including acute care, have been established in many schools of nursing.

EDUCATION

From 1965 until 1992, many NP programs were offered through schools of nursing in their continuing education departments. Programs were accredited by the American Nurses' Association (ANA), and graduates of NP programs could be certified by successfully passing an examination in any of the evolving NP specialties. The requirements for admission were few; the applicant had to be an RN, but graduates from diploma, associate degree, or higher programs were admitted if they had acceptable grades and scores in their previous course and clinical educational experiences. The guidelines for grant applications to the federal government stated that NP programs must be at least one academic year (nine months) long, with four months devoted to classroom and theoretical material, and five to six months to clinical practice time, with guidance and supervision from a physician or NP preceptor. NP preceptors were required to hold a master's degree and be certified in the specialty in which they were teaching/precepting. Most clinical practice occurred in primary care or community settings.

NONPF/ANA Guidelines

NP educators, through their respective schools and programs, formed the National Organization of Nurse Practitioner Faculties (NONPF) in the early 1970s. The purpose of the organization was to set both education and practice standards for NPs. In 1980, NONPF published *Guidelines for Family Nurse Practitioner Curricular Planning*, developed with funding from the Robert Wood Johnson Foundation. The guidelines were a major contribution to NP education. In subsequent years, NONPF published several additional guidelines, all of which present model program standards for NP education. NONPF's most recent publication is *Curriculum Guidelines and Program Standards for Nurse Practitioner Education* (1995).

The NONPF guidelines are based on particular assumptions regarding the role of NPs:[3]

1. Nurse practitioners are educated to practice both independently and interdependently. This practice includes cooperative and/or collaborative practice arrangements with other health care disciplines as members of interdisciplinary health care teams.
2. Nurse practitioners are accountable as *direct* providers of health care services.
3. The recipients of care by nurse practitioners, based on a population perspective, ideally includes individuals, families, and/or communities.

4. Clinical decision making based on critical thinking and diagnostic reasoning is fundamental to nurse practitioner practice.

5. Nurse practitioners are required to synthesize theoretical, scientific, and clinical knowledge as well as practice-based skills in the diagnosis and management of existing and potential health and illness states.

6. Health maintenance, health promotion, disease prevention, and health restoration are central goals of nurse practitioner care. Although the long-term goal of the nurse practitioners is to promote and restore health, short-term goals frequently include symptom or problem management. Each encounter is viewed as an opportunity to facilitate the client's movement toward health promotion, disease prevention, and restoration of health (high level health). If restoration of health is not possible, the nurse practitioner may support the client toward attaining the goal of a comfortable death.

7. Nurse practitioners provide cost-effective, coordinated, and comprehensive clinical care based on the best current knowledge of treatment outcomes. Strategies of care include advocacy for individuals and/or groups, decision making related to personal health, mobilization of resources, therapeutics (pharmacologic, nonpharmacologic, traditional, nontraditional), health education and counseling, coordination of services, and evaluation of treatment outcomes.

8. Nurse practitioners function in a variety of settings, using multiple practice models to improve treatment outcomes and coordination of services.

9. Nurse practitioners provide leadership in health care and in the nursing profession.

The 1995 NONPF publication states that the National League for Nursing (NLN) accreditation and evaluation standards have provided essential background standards for the development of NONPF's curriculum guidelines. An additional document, *Nursing's Social Policy Statement*, published by the ANA in 1995, includes four essential features of contemporary nursing practice. The statement defines nursing as "the diagnosis and treatment of human responses to actual or potential health problems," and lists as the essential components:[4]

- attention to the full range of human experiences and responses to health and illness without restriction to a problem-focused orientation;

- integration of objective data with knowledge gained from an understanding of the patient or group's subjective experience;
- application of scientific knowledge to the processes of diagnosis and treatment; and
- provision of a caring relationship that facilitates health and healing.

The policy statement adds:

> Nursing's scope of practice is dynamic and evolves with changes in the phenomena of concern, knowledge about the effects of various interventions on patient or group outcomes, the political environment, legal conditions, and cultural and demographic patterns of society. The scope of practice of nurses has a flexible boundary that is responsive to the changing needs of society. This boundary intersects with the scope of practices of other health professions.

The policy statement describes advanced nursing practice as the incorporation of

> specialization, expansion, and advancement in practice. Specialization is concentrating or delimiting one's focus to part of the whole field of nursing. Expansion refers to the acquisition of new practice knowledge and skills, particularly the knowledge and skills that legitimize role autonomy within the areas of practice that overlap traditional boundaries of medical practice. Advancement involves both specialization and expansion and is research-based, using practical knowledge that occurs as a part of graduate education in nursing.

NONPF curriculum guidelines are organized according to six domains of practice:

1. Management of client health/illness status
2. The nurse-client relationship
3. The teaching/coaching function
4. Professional role
5. Managing and negotiating health care delivery systems
6. Monitoring and ensuring the quality of health care practice

Specific competencies are listed under each domain, which are achieved as the NP student advances from the novice (beginner) phase, through advanced beginner, competent, proficient, and expert phases of growth in the individual's choice of practice area and level of expertise. *Competence* is defined as a level of performance; *competency* refers to a skilled nursing practice.

Academic Degree Programs

Gradually, individual schools began to set higher standards for admission to NP programs; at first, the Bachelor's degree in Science with specialty in Nursing (BSN) was required. The programs were then structured to be at master's degree level. In 1992, the ANA made the master's degree a requirement for graduates of NP programs to take the national certifying examination. Therefore, NP programs were offered only in colleges or universities that awarded master's degrees in nursing. Applicants who had a master's degree could enroll in post-master's-degree programs and take the courses and clinical experiences required for NP students; students did not have to repeat core courses that they had previously taken for the master's degree. In this way, many clinical nurse specialists (CNSs) have received their NP education and have been able to be certified as both CNSs and NPs.

The increased educational preparation of NPs paralleled the maturing of the NP role as an advanced practice nurse (APN). During the past 15 years, as NP programs have been mainstreamed within master's degree nursing programs, the foundation of core content, values, skills, and competencies needed by NPs to function, has been safeguarded.[3] The major thrust of the NP role was, and continues to be, built on a foundation of graduate education that allows NPs to function as clinicians in primary care settings and in specialty areas of practice, depending on education and students' choices.

The NP role is grounded in specialized theoretical knowledge and expanded practice skills in the areas of advanced clinical decision making, research, community organization, community and interdisciplinary collaboration, and leadership in all settings.[3]

Curriculum

A master's degree in nursing and completion of a graduate level program for preparation of NPs are required for national certification. NP programs should be a minimum of nine months (one academic year) of full-time study, or its equivalent, as defined by the sponsoring institution. About one-third of the program should be devoted to classroom or didactic experiences; the remaining two-thirds should be scheduled for clinical/preceptorship experiences. Teaching content and strategy should include, but not be limited to:

- A theory-based curriculum that uses scientific inquiry as the basis for advanced clinical practice
- A structural approach to teach skills in clinical reasoning (see Appendix A)
- A multidisciplinary approach
- The role of the consumer in health care
- The role of the professional in advanced practice
- The impact of health policy and organizational issues on health care
- The commitment to advancing clinical practice through research

The didactic component should feature a review and application of theories from the following physical and behavioral sciences:

- Anatomy and physiology
- Epidemiology
- Nursing and medical sciences
- Advanced pathophysiology
- Advanced pharmacology
- Social sciences

Epidemiology and genetics, rapidly expanding fields of knowledge that affect health, are currently in place in some schools or are expected to be added to core curriculums soon, as are courses in community health nursing.

Courses structured to teach decision making and clinical management process for adults should include:

Data-gathering techniques (interviewing, health history, physical and
    developmental assessment, family and social data)
Health promotion, education, and maintenance
Teaching, counseling, and anticipatory guidance for parents
Management of common acute and chronic health problems
Consultation and referral
Data management (computer-based medical records)
Ethical and legal considerations

Additional courses should include:

Research methods
    Participation
    Utilization
Professionalism in advanced practice
    Standards of practice
    Legal parameters of advanced practice

Credentialing
Quality assurance
Peer review
Prescriptive authority
Risk management
Professional organizations
Nurse practitioner role development
Historical perspective
Scope of practice
Multiple roles
Collaborative practice
Marketing
Political involvement
Health policy and organization issues
Access to care: primary care delivery, resource utilization, case management, policy research utilization/application, international health-care trends
Organizational management issues
Change strategies
Organizational communications, negotiations, legislative strategies, community involvement
Economics
Patient payment methods
Provider reimbursement mechanisms
Social programs

The clinical component of the program should provide supervised clinical and preceptorship experiences that include research utilization, assessment and management, technical and decision-making skills needed for optimal functioning as an adult NP, and assessment and diagnostic procedures.

FUNCTIONS OF NPs

On completion of a formal educational program, NPs are able to:

1. Elicit a comprehensive health history, including development, maturation, coping ability, activities of daily living, physiological functioning, and emotional and social well-being.
2. Perform a complete physical examination on adult patients.
3. Order and/or perform pertinent diagnostic tests.
4. Analyze the data collected to determine health status.

5. Formulate a problem list.
6. Develop and implement, with the patient, a plan of care to promote, maintain, and restore health.
7. Evaluate, with the patient, the patient's response to the health care provided and the effectiveness of the care.
8. Modify the health-care plan and intervention/treatment as needed.
9. Collaborate with other health-care professionals in meeting patients' health-care needs.
10. Record all pertinent data about the patient, including history and physical examination findings, problems identified, interventions provided, results of care, and plan for follow-up or referral as appropriate.
11. Coordinate the services required to meet patients' needs for health care.
12. Define the adult NP role and the scope of practice for the primary health care.
13. Identify and implement strategies to maximize the role of the CANP.
14. Develop and implement strategies that have a positive effect on the political and regulatory processes related to health-care systems and to the role of the CANP.

The Maryland Nurse Practice Act for NPs is reprinted in Appendix B for the reader's general reference and information.

SPECIALTIES

NP specialties are currently being offered in master's degree programs by 206 universities. The total number of NP programs available is 483, because many schools of nursing offer several NP specialties. The number and percentage of programs are shown in Table 5-1.

Family Nurse Practitioner

An FNP is an RN with a graduate degree in nursing who is prepared for advanced practice with individuals and families throughout the patient's life span and across the health continuum. FNP practice includes independent and interdependent decision making and direct accountability for clinical judgment.

Most master's degree programs to prepare FNPs are at least three semesters long, and many require two years to complete the program. The

TABLE 5–1
Master's degree programs for NPs

Type of Specialty	No. of Programs	% of Programs
Family	143	77.7
Pediatric	64	34.8
Gerontological	51	27.7
Adult	49	26.6
Ob/Gyn/Women's Health	47	25.5
Neonatal	33	17.9
Adult Psychiatric/Mental Health	23	12.5
Adult Acute Care	22	11.9
Oncology	9	4.9
Occupational Health	8	4.3
School	6	3.3
Child and Adolescent Psychiatric/ Mental Health	5	2.7
Perinatal	5	2.7
Other, including dual-track options	18	9.8

Source: Data from American Association of Colleges of Nursing, 1995. Proceedings of the Master's Education Conference, San Antonio, TX, December 8–10, 1994.

didactic content and clinical preceptorship ratio of 1:2 is the same as described for NPs. Didactic content for NPs includes material regarding patients from birth to old age and for both men and women. The clinical experiences include managing the care of patients with acute and chronic health problems in all age groups.

The scope of practice of FNPs is greater than that for other APN specialties, and the demand for the services of FNPs is also higher because of their capability of caring for all family members.

School Nurse Practitioner

School NPs are RNs prepared in formal educational programs to assume responsibilities in the health care of preschool and school-age children, and adolescents. The practice requires knowledge of educational systems, school health, community health, health education, and planning for the needs of exceptional children and their parents. In addition, school NPs have specific functions:

- Perform age-appropriate developmental evaluations to assess normal and abnormal variations of motor, cognitive, social, emotional, and perceptual aspects of child development.
- Perform pertinent screening measures to determine health status.
- Collaborate with teachers, school personnel, community agencies, and other health care professionals to meet health care needs.
- Provide health education to individuals and groups, using methods designed to increase individuals' motivation and ability to assume responsibility for their own health care.
- Provide guidance to teachers and parents regarding recognition of child abuse and its reporting and prevention, environmental concerns (such as lead poisoning), eating disorders, safety promotion, and adolescent health issues.

Certified Pediatric Nurse Practitioner

CPNPs are RNs prepared at the graduate level to assume a role as a principal provider of primary health care for children. Pediatric NPs provide direct and indirect nursing services to children and their families in specific areas of health promotion, health maintenance, and health restoration.

The educational program to prepare pediatric NPs is similar to that of the school NP.

Gerontological Nurse Practitioner

GNPs are experts in providing primary health care for older adults and their families in a variety of settings. In providing care and advocacy for the older adult, these NPs work to maximize functional abilities; promote, maintain, and restore health; prevent or minimize disabilities; and assist the dying person to have dignity and autonomy to the degree possible, for as long as possible.

The functions of the GNP are much the same as those of the CANP, except that the focus is on the older adult who generally has more complex health problems than do younger persons. The GNP has increased awareness of special problems that occur in older persons: elder abuse and neglect, pharmacodynamics and pharmacokinetics, environmental hazards, decreased hearing and speech capabilities, and symptoms of illness that may not be as pronounced or evident as they may be in younger persons. The GNP helps the family to cope with the daily care of the older person and incorporates assistance from community and other agencies to maximize care.

Women's Health Care Nurse Practitioner

The focus of care provided by women's health care NPs is the particular problems of women of all ages, including normal development; life stages in the reproductive, menopausal, and postmenopausal years; fertility and infertility problems; family planning; prenatal and postpartum care; and acute and chronic problems that particularly occur in women.

Neonatal Nurse Practitioner

The neonatal NP works almost exclusively in acute care settings, primarily in hospital neonatal intensive care units. Program requirements include 200 hours of didactic/theoretical content and at least 600 hours in clinical/ preceptorship practice. Eligibility to take the certification examination requires 2000 hours and two years' experience in neonatal intensive care nursing.

Acute Care Nurse Practitioner

An acute care nurse practitioner (ACNP) is an RN with a graduate degree in nursing who is prepared for advanced practice in acute care. This practice, using a collaborative model, includes the provision of direct services to patients who are acutely or critically ill in a variety of settings. Diagnostic reasoning, advanced therapeutic interventions, and education are key elements in the direct provision of care by the ACNP. The ACNP also uses skills in consultation, collaboration, and systems management in providing effective restorative care. The practice of the ACNP includes independent and interdependent decision making and direct accountability for clinical judgment.

About 25 schools of nursing have already developed ACNP programs in anticipation of increasing demands for NPs prepared in this specialty. The acute care setting is different traditionally from the major purpose for which NPs were educated—to practice in primary care. In recent years, however, NPs who have been hired by hospitals have been so effective that the demand has skyrocketed.

CERTIFICATION

NPs may become certified by taking national certification examinations in any of the specialties, depending on their educational preparation.

NPs are certified through the American Nurses' Credentialing Center (ANCC), an arm of the ANA; the National Certification Boards of Pediatric Nurse Practitioners and Nurses; and the National Certification Corporation for the Obstetric, Gynecologic, and Neonatal Nurse Specialties (NCC). Many states also provide certification by means of recognition processes.

Women's Health Care NP

The certification examination taken by graduates of Women's Health Care NP master's programs include questions in the following categories: (1) general health (20–25%), (2) gynecology (40–45%), and (3) obstetrics (35–40%).

Neonatal NP

The certification examination includes questions in the following areas: (1) general assessment (15–20%); (2) general management (20–25%); (3) disease processes—embryology, physiology, and pathophysiology of all body systems (55–60%); (4) family integration (less than 5%); and (5) professional issues (less than 5%).[5]

Acute Care NP

The ANCC developed the ACNP national certifying examination, together with qualifications and eligibility requirements, in response to hospitals' demand for NPs. The certification examination for ACNPs was offered for the first time in December 1995.

Applicants are eligible to take the certification examination if they have completed a master's degree program as an ACNP. From 1995 until the year 2000, CANPs may also sit for the examination if they can document having a minimum of 500 hours of practice over the previous two years in an advanced practice role, providing direct services to patients who are acutely or critically ill. Topics covered in the examination include system-specific health problems, common problems in acute care, professionalism in advanced practice, issues and trends, health promotion, and risk assessment.

SUMMARY

Education for NPs is rigorous and is audited by professional organizations and national certifying examinations, which are required in most states.

The primary purpose of rigid preparation and continuing education required for recertification every five years is to ensure the safety of patients who come under the care and guidance of NPs. As a group, NPs are committed to quality care and the health of their patients.

REFERENCES

1. American Nurses Credentialing Center. *1996 Certification Catalog*. Washington, DC: American Nurses Credentialing Center, 1996.
2. Ford, LC, Silver, HK. The expanded role of the nurse in child care. *Nursing Outlook*, 15(9):43–45, 1967.
3. National Organization of Nurse Practitioner Faculties. *Curriculum Guidelines and Program Standards for Nurse Practitioner Education*, 2nd ed. Washington, DC: National Organization of Nurse Practitioner Faculties, 1995.
4. American Nurses' Association. *Nursing's Social Policy Statement*. Washington, DC: American Nurses' Association, 1995.
5. National Certification Corporation for the Obstetric, Gynecologic and Neonatal Nursing Specialties. *1966 Certification Catalog*. Chicago: National Certification Corporation, 1996.

BIBLIOGRAPHY

Accreditation Committee, Council of Baccalaureate and Higher Degree Programs. *Criteria and Guidelines for the Evaluation of Baccalaureate and Higher Degree Programs in Nursing* (Publication No. 15-2474). New York: National League for Nursing Press, 1992.

McGivern DO. The evolution to advanced practice. In Mezey MO, McGivern DO, eds., *Nurses, Nurse Practitioners: Evolution to Advanced Practice*. New York: Springer, 1993.

Sultz HA, et al. *Longitudinal Study of Nurse Practitioners*: Phase I (1976), Phase II (1978), Phase III (1980). Washington DC: Department of Health, Education, and Welfare. No. 76-43 (Phase I), No. 78-92 (Phase II), No. HRA-80-2 (Phase III), 1980.

Sultz H, et al. A decade of change for NPs: Part I. *Nurs Outlook*, 31:137–142, 216–219, 1983.

Chapter 6

Nurse-Midwifery

HISTORY

Midwifery is an ancient art, based on the needs of women throughout history. Nurse-midwifery developed in the early part of the twentieth century as a particular nursing specialty, largely influenced by the work of Mary Breckenridge, an English-trained nurse-midwife who emigrated to the United States in the early 1920s and developed the Frontier Nursing Service in rural Kentucky. The service provided nursing and obstetric care to Scottish, English, and Welsh families who had settled in that rural Appalachian area as farmers, lumberers, and miners. Access to health care for these people was difficult, often requiring travel by crude methods over long distances to the nearest physician's office or hospital. The Frontier Nursing Service became a major source of primary care for these families, who numbered in the hundreds. The nurses traveled by horseback to the homes of women in labor, to patients with emergency illness or accident, and they provided expert care, teaching, and continuing support over many years. Programs of nurse-midwifery modeled after the Frontier Nursing Service developed across the United States, primarily as continuing education (nondegree) programs associated with schools of medicine or nursing. Two early programs were developed in the mid-1930s, one at Kings County Hospital in Brooklyn, New York, under the direction and support of Louis Hellman, MD, then the chief of obstetrics and gynecology at the hospital; the other at Roosevelt Hospital in Manhattan (known as the Maternity Center.)

Today, certified nurse-midwives (CNMs), educated mainly in master's-degree nursing programs, provide primary, obstetric, and infant care to thousands of women and children in all states and territories. They practice in free-standing birth centers, in collaborative private practices with obstetricians/gynecologists, in hospitals teamed with obstetricians/gynecologists or as a separate department, in their own private or CNM group practices, in health departments, and community clinics.

Most of the rest of this chapter contains information quoted directly from American College of Nurse-Midwives (ACNM) publications, which are available through their office in Washington, DC.*

DEFINITIONS

Nurse-Midwifery Practice

Nurse-midwifery practice is the independent management of women's health care, focusing particularly on pregnancy, childbirth, the postpartum period, care of the newborn, and the family planning and gynecological needs of women. The CNM practices within a health-care system that provides for consultation, collaborative management or referral as indicated by the health status of the client. CNMs practice in accord with the *Standards for the Practice of Nurse-Midwifery*, as defined by the American College of Nurse-Midwives.[1]

Certified Nurse-Midwife

A CNM is an individual educated in the two disciplines of nursing and midwifery, who possesses evidence of certification according to the requirements of the ACNM.[2] CNMs are educated in both master's and certificate (continuing education) nursing programs and provide primary, obstetric, infant, and well-women care to thousands of women and children. Primary care by CNMs includes preconception counseling, care during pregnancy and childbirth, provision of gynecological and contraceptive services, and care of the peri- and post-menopausal woman. With health education as a major focus, the goals are to prevent problems and to assist women in developing and maintaining healthy habits.[3]

Over the last decade, CNMs have extended their practice to include primary care to women throughout the life span. They provide care on a continuous and comprehensive basis by establishing a plan of

---

*Adapted and/or used in their entirety with permission of the ACNM.

management with the woman for her ongoing health care. The care is inclusive and is integrated with the cultural, socioeconomic, and psychological factors that may impinge on the woman's health status.[3]

CODE OF ETHICS

A CNM has professional moral obligations. The purpose of the code of ethics is to identify obligations that guide the CNM in the practice of nurse-midwifery. The code further serves to clarify the expectations of the profession to consumers, the public, other professionals and potential practitioners. The ACNM Code of Ethics states the following:[4]

1. Nurse-midwifery exists for the good of women and their families. This good is safeguarded by practice in accordance with the ACNM Philosophy and ACNM standards for the Practice of Nurse-Midwifery.
2. Nurse-midwives uphold the belief that childbearing and maturation are normal life processes. When intervention is indicated, it is integrated into care in a way that preserves the dignity of the woman and her family.
3. Decisions regarding nurse-midwifery care require client participation in an ongoing negotiation process in order to develop a safe plan of care. This process considers cultural diversity, individual autonomy, and legal responsibilities.
4. Nurse-midwives share professional information with their clients that leads to informed participation and consent. This sharing is done without coercion or deception.
5. Nurse-midwives practice competently. They consult and refer when indicated by their professional scope of practice and/or personal limitations.
6. Nurse-midwives provide care without discrimination based on race, religion, life-style, sexual orientation, socioeconomic status, or nature of health problem.
7. Nurse-midwives maintain confidentiality except when there is a clear, serious and immediate danger or when mandated by law.
8. Nurse-midwives take appropriate action to protect clients from harm when endangered by incompetent or unethical practices.
9. Nurse-midwives interact respectfully with the people with whom they work and practice.
10. Nurse-midwives participate in developing and improving the care of women and families through supporting the profession of nurse-midwifery, research, and the education of nurse-midwifery students and nurse-midwives.

11. Nurse-midwives promote community, state, and national efforts such as public education and legislation, to ensure access to quality care and to meet the health needs of women and their families.

EDUCATION/CERTIFICATION

The ACNM states that the preparation of nurse-midwives is uniform, regardless of where the education takes place, and does not require a master's degree for certification as a CNM as long as the education occurs under the ACNM curricular (competency) guidelines and under the aegis of the ACNM. The ACNM administers the certification examination taken by all graduates of CNM programs, which therefore ensures that all CNMs are prepared at the same level to perform at the professional level. All CNM education programs are affiliated with an institution of higher learning and have standardized criteria for ACNM accreditation and a standardized curriculum.[5]

The ACNM adopted its articles of incorporation and bylaws in 1955. The objectives of the organization relate primarily to standards of education and practice of CNMs. The ACNM's *Articles of Incorporation and Bylaws,* amended through May 1995, include objectives and are available from the ACNM.*

ACNM Philosophy

CNMs believe that every individual has the right to safe, satisfying health care, with respect for human dignity and cultural variations, and support each person's right to self-determination, to complete information, and to active participation in all aspects of care. CNMs believe the normal processes of pregnancy and birth can be enhanced through education, health care, and supportive intervention.[6] The philosophy statement continues:

> Nurse-midwifery care is focused on the needs of the individual and family for physical care, emotional and social support, and active involvement of significant others according to cultural values and personal preferences. The practice of nurse-midwifery encourages continuity of care; emphasizes safe, competent clinical management; advocates nonintervention in normal processes; and promotes health education for women throughout the childbearing cycle. This practice may extend to include gynecological care of well women throughout the life cycle. Such comprehensive health care is most effectively and efficiently provided by [CNMs] in collaboration with other members of an interdependent health-care team.

---

*ACNM, 818 Connecticut Ave. N.W., Suite 900, Washington, DC 20006 (202-728-9860).

The ACNM assumes a leadership role in the development and promotion of high-quality health care for women and infants both nationally and internationally. The profession of nurse-midwifery is committed to ensuring that certified nurse-midwives are provided with sound educational preparation, to expanding knowledge through research, and to evaluating and revising care through quality assurance. The profession further ensures that its members adhere to its Standards of Practice for Nurse-Midwifery in accordance with the ACNM philosophy.[6]

ACNM Mission Statement

The mission statement of the ACNM declares that its purpose is "[t]o develop and support the profession of nurse-midwifery in order to promote the health and well-being of women and infants within their families and communities."[5]

BASIC CORE COMPETENCIES

Nurse-midwifery education is based on theoretical preparation in the sciences and clinical preparation for the judgment and skills necessary for management of the care of women and newborns. The care as defined by the ACNM includes antepartum, intrapartum, postpartum, neonatal, family planning, and well-woman gynecology, and occurs within a health-care system that provides for collaboration (co-management) and referral. Nurse-midwifery practice is based on these Core Competencies, the Standards for the Practice of Nurse-Midwifery, and the ACNM Code of Ethics. CNMs assume responsibility and accountability for practice by applying their knowledge and skills in a process for clinical decision making: the management process. The 1993 ACNM publication continues:[7]

Core competencies delineate the fundamental knowledge, skills, and behaviors expected of a new graduate. Because nurse-midwifery practice continues to be a dynamic and changing discipline, these core competencies are presented as guidelines only for educators, students, physicians and other professionals, consumers, and employers of nurse-midwives. The guidelines will continue to evolve with the practice of nurse-midwifery. The concepts and skills identified . . . below and the aspects of the nurse-midwifery management process [here] apply to all components of nurse-midwifery care. . . .

Because creativity and individuality in nurse-midwifery education are essential to the vitality of the profession, educational programs are encouraged to be innovative. Each program will develop its own characteristics and may extend into other areas of health care. Each graduate is responsible for practicing in accordance with state laws and institutional protocols. Core competencies remain, however, as the basic requisites for the graduate of any educational program.

Certain concepts and skills from the social sciences and public health permeate all aspects of nurse-midwifery practice. The following have been identified:

1. Promotion of family-centered care.
2. Facilitation of healthy family and interpersonal relationships.
3. Constructive use of communication and of guidance and counseling skills.
4. Communication and collaboration with other members of the health team.
5. Provision of health education.
6. Promotion of continuity of care.
7. Use of appropriate community resources.
8. Promotion of health and prevention of disease throughout the life cycle.
9. Recognition of pregnancy as a normal physiologic and development process.
10. Advocacy for informed choice and decision making.
11. Consideration of bioethical issues related to women's health.
12. Knowledge of and respect for cultural variations.

Skills Beyond Basic Competencies

To be eligible to take the Certification Council examination, the CNM candidate must demonstrate scientific knowledge and clinical skills as outlined by the *ACNM Core Competencies for Basic Nurse-Midwifery Practice*. "As science and technology advance to create changes in health-care delivery, CNMs will be required to possess knowledge and skills beyond the basic level of nurse-midwifery practice. Specialization in particular areas may further define an individual's practice."[8] The *Expansion* of core competencies publication goes on to say:

[To ensure] that new technical skills remain within the scope and safety of nurse-midwifery practice, the ACNM requires that the incorporation of these skills be accomplished in accordance with the current Standards for the Practice of Nurse-Midwifery and [the ACNM] *Guidelines for the Incorporation of New Procedures into Nurse-Midwifery Practice*,[9] including proper documentation of the process of incorporating new technical skills.

Mandatory Degree Requirements for Nurse-Midwives

The ACNM supports educational programs for CNMs at both certificate and degree levels, and opposes mandatory degree requirements for state licensure for CNMs.[10]

> The safety and quality of entry-level nurse-midwifery practice is [en]sured by the ACNM Certification Council, whose testing and certification procedures have been recognized by the National Commission of Health Certifying Agencies and by the ACNM Division of Accreditation, an accrediting body recognized by the U.S. Department of Education, which [en]sures the quality and content of nurse-midwifery education programs.

> Differences in nurse-midwifery educational background have not resulted in differences in certification test results. Analysis of certification examination results demonstrates that academic degrees do not enhance the clinical competence of a nurse-midwife; both certificate and degree programs prepare competent, beginning CNMs. However, pursuit of higher degrees by CNMs is encouraged for the purpose of preparing educators, researchers, and theoreticians because these roles are important for advancing the profession.

> The ACNM believes that mandatory degree requirements limit access to maternity and gynecological services by denying practice opportunities for CNMs in states in which academic degrees are mandatory. "Several national reports specifically recommend placing greater reliance on CNMs to increase access to prenatal care for underserved populations. These reports also recommend that state laws should be supportive of nurse-midwifery practice."[10]

HEALTH-CARE RESPONSIBILITIES

Client Health-Care Management

Nurse-midwifery management of care has three aspects: primary management, collaborative management (co-management), and referral management. Implicit in this process is timely action and the documentation of all its aspects.[7] The responsibilities of the CNM in each aspect of management, as defined by the ACNM in *Core Competencies for Basic Nurse-Midwifery Practice*,[7] are presented in Table 6–1.

TABLE 6–1
Certified nurse-midwifery management core competencies

I. Primary Management

A. Systematically obtains or updates a complete and relevant data base for assessment of the client's health status.

B. Accurately identifies problems and diagnoses based on correct interpretations of the data base.

C. Delineates health-care goals and formulates and communicates a complete needs/problems list in collaboration with the woman.

D. Identifies need for consultation with or referral to appropriate members of the health-care team.

E. Provides information and support to enable women to make appropriate decisions and to assume appropriate responsibility for their own health.

F. Develops a comprehensive plan of care with the woman based on supportive rationale.

G. Assumes direct responsibility for implementing the plan of care.

H. Initiates management of deviation from normal, including emergencies and specific complications.

I. Evaluates, with the woman, the achievement of health-care goals and modifies the plan of care accordingly.

II. Collaboration (Co-Management)

A. Identifies problems and related complications requiring consultation and collaboration (co-management).

B. Obtains consultation; plans and implements collaborative management (co-management) with other providers.

C. Continues management of midwifery aspects of care.

D. Serves as consultant or co-manager for other providers.

III. Referral

A. Identifies the need for comprehensive management and care outside the scope of practice.

B. Selects appropriate sources of care in collaboration with the woman.

C. Transfers the care of the client as appropriate.

Source: Board of Directors, American College of Nurse-Midwives. *ACNM Core Competencies for Basic Nurse-Midwifery Practice.* Washington, DC: American College of Nurse-Midwives, May 1985 (rev. Feb. 1992). Used with permission.

Skills for Areas of Practice

Implicit in a nurse-midwifery knowledge base is the ability to perform skills pertinent to each of the outlined areas of practice[7] shown in Table 6–2.

TABLE 6–2
Components of nurse-midwifery care

I. *Preconception Care*

A. Assumes responsibility for management of care of the woman who is preparing for pregnancy.
B. Uses a foundation for nurse-midwifery practice that includes but is not limited to the knowledge of:
    1. Female and male reproductive anatomy and physiology related to conception.
    2. Health history, family history, and relevant genetic history.
    3. Health and laboratory screening to evaluate the potential for a healthy pregnancy.
    4. Assessment of emotional, psychosocial, sexual status, and readiness for pregnancy of the woman and her support system.
    5. Nutritional assessment and counseling.
    6. Influence of environmental and occupational factors, health habits, and behavior on pregnancy planning.

II. *Antepartum Care*

A. Assumes responsibility for management of care of the pregnant woman.
B. Uses a foundation for nurse-midwifery practice that includes but is not limited to the knowledge of:
    1. Female anatomy and physiology.
    2. Anatomy and physiology of conception, pregnancy, and lactation.
    3. Clinical application of genetics, embryology, and fetal development.
    4. Diagnosis of pregnancy.
    5. Assessment of the woman's emotional status and her support systems.
    6. Common screening/diagnostic tests used during pregnancy.
    7. Indicators of normal pregnancy.
    8. Causes of maternal morbidity and mortality.
    9. Indicators of risk and complications in pregnancy and appropriate interventions.
    10. Parameters and methods for assessing the progress of pregnancy.
    11. Parameters and methods for assessing fetal well-being.
    12. Nutritional assessment and counseling of the pregnant woman.
    13. The influence of environmental and occupational factors, health habits, and maternal behaviors on the family.

TABLE 6–2 *Continued*

14. The etiology and management of common discomforts of pregnancy.
15. Pharmacokinetics of medications commonly used during pregnancy.
16. Prescription of medications and treatments.
17. Psychosocial, emotional, sexual changes during pregnancy.
18. Planning and implementation of individual and/or group education.
19. Counseling on the physical and emotional changes of pregnancy, preparation for birth, lactation, parenthood, and change in the family constellation.

III. Intrapartum Care

A. Assumes responsibility for management of care of the woman and fetus during the intrapartum period.
B. Uses a foundation for nurse-midwifery practice that includes but is not limited to the knowledge of:
   1. Anatomy and physiology of normal and abnormal labor processes through the four stages.
   2. Anatomy of the fetal skull and its critical landmarks.
   3. Parameters and methods for assessing progress of labor through the four stages.
   4. Parameters and methods for assessing maternal and fetal status.
   5. Common screening/diagnostic tests used during labor.
   6. Emotional changes during labor and delivery.
   7. Physical and emotional support measures used during labor and birth.
   8. Pharmacokinetics of medications commonly used during labor and birth, including effects on mother and fetus.
   9. Prescription or administration of appropriate medications and solutions during labor and birth.
   10. Techniques for administration of local and pundendal anesthesia.
   11. Techniques for spontaneous vaginal delivery.
   12. Indicators of deviations from normal and appropriate interventions.
   13. Diagnosis and assessment of labor and its progress through the four stages.
   14. Techniques for management of abnormal birth events.
   15. Anatomy, physiology, and indicators of normal adaptation of newborn to extrauterine life.
   16. Techniques for placental expulsion.
   17. Techniques for performance and repair of episiotomy and repair of lacerations.

IV. Postpartum Care

A. Assumes responsibility for management of care of the woman during the postpartum period.

Continued

TABLE 6–2   *Continued*

B. Uses a foundation for nurse-midwifery practice that includes but is not
limited to the knowledge of:
1. Anatomy and physiology of the puerperium, including the involutional
process.
2. Anatomy and physiology of lactation and methods for its facilitation or
suppression.
3. Parameters and methods for assessing the puerperium.
4. Emotional, psychosocial, and sexual changes of the puerperium.
5. Etiology and methods for managing discomforts of the puerperium.
6. Common screening/diagnostic tests used during the puerperium.
7. Indicators of deviations from normal and appropriate interventions.
8. Pharmacokinetics of medications commonly used during the
puerperium.
9. Prescription or administration of appropriate medications, treatments,
and solutions.
10. Appropriate anticipatory guidance regarding self-care, infant care,
family planning, and family relationships.

V. Neonatal Care

A. Assumes responsibility for management of care of the neonate.
B. Uses a foundation for nurse-midwifery practice that includes but is not
limited to the knowledge of:
1. Anatomy and physiology of adaptation to extrauterine life and
stabilization of the neonate.
2. Parameters and methods for assessing neonatal status, including
emotional and psychosocial needs.
3. Parameters and methods for assessing gestational age of the neonate.
4. Nutritional needs of the neonate.
5. Indicators of deviations from normal and appropriate intervention.
6. Screening/diagnostic tests performed on the neonate.
7. Pharmacokinetics of medications commonly used for the neonate.
8. Prescription of medications and treatments.
9. Methods to facilitate adaptation to extrauterine life including
resuscitation and emergency care of the newborn.
10. Factors influencing neonatal behavior and parental interaction.

IV. Family Planning/Gynecological Care

A. Assumes responsibility for management of care of women seeking family
planning and/or gynecologic services.
B. Uses a foundation for nurse-midwifery practice that includes but is not
limited to the knowledge of:
1. Anatomy and physiology of the reproductive system through the
life cycle.
2. Anatomy and physiology of the female breast.

TABLE 6–2 *Continued*

---

3. Anatomy, physiology, and psychosocial components of human sexuality.
4. Provision of counseling regarding general health promotion.
5. Common screening and diagnostic tests.
6. Factors relating to barrier, steroidal, mechanical, chemical, physiologic, and surgical conception control methods, including:
   a. Rationale for use
   b. Contraindications to use
   c. Effectiveness rates
   d. Mechanisms of action
   e. Advantages/disadvantages
   f. Risks/side effects/complications
   g. Comparative cost
   h. Instruction/counseling
   i. Psychological and sexual considerations
   j. Provision of appropriate method
   k. Discontinuation or change of method
7. Indicators of developmental changes of women throughout the life cycle and health promotion measures specific to these changes.
8. Indicators of problems of sexuality, methods for counseling, and indications for consultation or referral.
9. Factors involved in decision making regarding unplanned or undesired pregnancies and resources for counseling and referral.
10. Indicators of deviations from normal, risk factors, and appropriate preventive measures and interventions for selected pathology.

Source: Board of Directors, American College of Nurse-Midwives. *ACNM Core Competencies for Basic Nurse-Midwifery Practice.* Washington, DC: American College of Nurse-Midwives, May 1985 (rev. Feb. 1992). Used with permission.

PROFESSIONAL RESPONSIBILITIES

The CNM assumes the role and professional responsibilities of nurse-midwifery practice as defined by the ACNM. As a leader or change agent, the nurse-midwife demonstrates:[7]

1. Knowledge of the historical development of nurse-midwifery in the United States, the structure and function of the ACNM, and the legal base for nurse-midwifery practice.
2. Knowledge of contemporary issues and trends in maternal-child health care nationally and internationally.
3. Knowledge of standards for quality maternal and child health services.

4. Knowledge of current and pending health legislation.
5. Knowledge of the role and responsibilities of the CNM in supporting legislative contributions to high-quality maternal and child health services.
6. Knowledge of the various nurse-midwifery practice options and the resources available for their development and evaluation.
7. The ability to carry out the philosophy of the ACNM.
8. Respect for the dignity and rights of health-care providers and clients.
9. Responsibility and accountability for:
   a. Personal management decisions made in caring for clients.
   b. Periodic self-evaluation and participation in peer review to maintain currency in practice.
   c. Delivery of services to families in collaboration with other health care providers.
10. The ability to evaluate, apply, and collaborate in research.
11. Awareness of the professional responsibility to participate in nurse-midwifery education.

CERTIFIED NURSE-MIDWIVES IN MARYLAND

There are 225 CNMs in Maryland. In particular cities the numbers are: metropolitan District of Columbia—19; Baltimore—35; Salisbury—6; Frederick—7. Practice by CNMs occurs in many settings, throughout the state, for example, hospitals, clinics, health maintenance organizations (HMOs), private homes, birth centers, and private practices. Thirty-five nurse-midwifery practice sites are located across the state.

In 1990, CNMs provided a total of 34,900 (31%) of 112,600 prenatal public health contacts in Maryland. In 1992, CNMs attended 4,038 births of which 3,630 occurred in hospitals, 388 in birth centers, and 30 in homes.

Two freestanding birth centers are located in Maryland. Both received the 1991 Annual Leadership Award for Innovative Health Programs from the Foundation for Nursing of Maryland, Inc. CNMs receive full reimbursement from third-party payers for their services. In July 1990, CNMs in Maryland obtained prescriptive privileges.[11] The Maryland Nurse Practice Act for CNMs is reprinted in Appendix C for the reader's general reference and information.

REFERENCES

1. Board of Directors, American College of Nurse-Midwives. *Definition of Nurse-Midwifery Practice.* Washington, DC: American College of Nurse-Midwives, July 1992 (rev. Aug. 1993).
2. ———. *Definition of a Certified Nurse-Midwife.* Washington, DC. American College of Nurse-Midwives, Jan. 1978 (rev. Aug. 1993).
3. ———. *Certified Nurse-Midwives as Primary Care Providers.* Washington, DC: American College of Nurse-Midwives, Oct. 1992 (rev. Nov. 1994).
4. ———. *Code of Ethics for Certified Nurse-Midwives.* Washington, DC: American College of Nurse-Midwives, May 1990 (rev. Nov. 1994).
5. ———. *ACNM Mission Statement.* Washington, DC: American College of Nurse-Midwives, Oct. 1992.
6. ———. *Philosophy of the ACNM.* Washington, DC: American College of Nurse-Midwives, Oct. 1989.
7. ———. *ACNM Core Competencies for Basic Nurse-Midwifery Practice.* Washington, DC: American College of Nurse-Midwives, May 1985 (rev. Feb. 1992).
8. ———. *Expansion of Nurse-Midwifery Practice and Skills Beyond Basic Core Competencies.* Washington, DC: American College of Nurse-Midwives, July 1992.
9. ———. *Guidelines for the Incorporation of New Procedures into Nurse-Midwifery Practice.* Washington, DC: American College of Nurse-Midwives, July 1992.
10. Division of Accreditation/Education Committee, American College of Nurse-Midwives. *Mandatory Degree Requirements for Nurse-Midwives.* Washington, DC: American College of Nurse-Midwives, 1992, 1994.
11. Data for Maryland from ACNM, *Certified Nurse-Midwives in Maryland* (PR 94, 12/19); and D. Williams, Director of Professional Services and Support, American College of Nurse-Midwives. Personal communication, 1995.

BIBLIOGRAPHY

Board of Directors, American College of Nurse-Midwives. *Continuing Competency Assessment.* Washington, DC: American College of Nurse-Midwives, May 1992.
———. *Nurse-Midwifery Education.* Washington, DC: American College of Nurse-Midwives, Nov. 1992 (rev. Nov. 1994).
———. *Standards for the Practice of Nurse-Midwifery.* Washington, DC: American College of Nurse-Midwives, 1992.
———. *Nurse-Midwifery Education.* Washington, DC: American College of Nurse-Midwives, Oct. 1994.
Joint Statement of MANA and ACNM. *Midwifery Certification in the United States.* Washington, DC: American College of Nurse-Midwives, April 1993.

Joint Statement of Practice Relations Between Obstetrician/Gynecologist and Certified Nurse-Midwives. Washington, DC: American College of Nurse-Midwives, Nov. 1992 (rev. 1994).

National Commission of Nurse-Midwifery Education. *Educating Nurse-Midwives: A Strategy for Achieving Affordable, High-Quality Maternity Care.* Washington, DC: American College of Nurse-Midwives, 1993.

Varney, H. *Nurse-Midwifery,* 2nd ed. Boston: Blackwell Scientific, 1987.

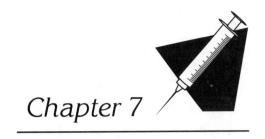

Chapter 7

Clinical Nurse Specialist

History
Definition
Responsibilities
Education/Certification
Specialties
Summary

Clinical nurse specialists (CNSs) have been educated at the master's-degree level since the specialty began in the mid to late 1960s, about the same time as nurse practitioner (NP) programs began. The practice of the CNS is within the domain of nursing and does not usually overlap the domain of medicine as does the practice of an NP, a CNM, and a CRNA, except for the psychiatric CNS, who provides diagnostic, counseling, and psychiatric services, which sometimes do overlap with the services and treatment provided by physician psychiatrists. Nevertheless, many CNSs, by virtue of extensive experience and position requirements, become proficient at performing comprehensive physical assessments and diagnosing disease states occurring in patients; thus, they may provide medical care, albeit usually under the direction and guidance of physicians.

HISTORY

In the decades following World War II, with the proliferation of medical, surgical, pediatric, and neonatal intensive care units, cardiac surgery, and special needs of physically and mentally severely ill patients in hospitals, nursing leaders saw the need for more highly educated and specialized nurses. Reiter and Peplau were among the early proponents of CNSs, as this group of nurses came to be known. In 1954, Hildegard Peplau developed the first master's-degree program in psychiatric nursing at Rutgers University. Many nurse educators credit Peplau's work as the major driving force for education of clinical specialists at the master's degree level. Master's degree programs for nurses were developing rapidly during this period, aided in large part by federal funds through the GI Bill and for construction of nursing schools to meet the growing demand and evident need for highly educated nurses. The graduate degree was considered essential for the CNS to function in specialized roles. Through master's degree programs, CNSs obtained not only additional technical knowledge, but also "a theoretical background in the various sciences which contributed to the CNSs' clinical practice expertise, and to the profession of nursing as an applied science."[1] Master's degree education included systematic, supervised clinical experience; seminars focused on clinical and professional problems; research methodology; biostatistics; and other areas of science.

> Master's education prepared the CNS to (a) identify systematically and accurately the nursing needs of patients; (b) devise and implement appropriate clinical nursing plans for individual patients; (c) make observational studies of patient needs and evaluate nursing requirements; (d) translate research findings into actual nursing practice; (e) institute patient care improvements; (f) serve as a "model" of expert clinical nursing to other nursing personnel; and (g) generally serve as a resource of clinical nursing expertise to the staff of the unit.[1]

Nursing expertise was defined as representing knowledge drawn from the biological, social, and medical sciences and codified into nursing knowledge. Examples of expertise are: (1) knowledge of how respiratory and circulatory systems function under stress; (2) awareness of circumstances in which patients are likely to conceal or deny anxiety; (3) understanding of ethnic or class variables that affect a patient's responsibilities for self-care after discharge from the hospital; (4) understanding ways in which the bureaucratic regulatory procedures on the unit may be extended to meet particular patient problems; and (5) scientific knowledge of the diagnostic warning signs of impending physical crises in patients (e.g., pulmonary embolism, shock, diabetic coma); and (6) similar other aspects of nursing practice.

This era therefore marked the beginning of systematic scientific education, practice, and research for nurses. The greatest need for specialized nurses at this time was seen in the area of psychiatry, particularly because of the large number of servicemen suffering from various types of mental disorders caused by their experiences in war. Servicemen with psychiatric problems filled both military and public hospital units; the need for nurses with expert knowledge about psychiatric problems was enormous. The

1946 National Mental Health Act provided federal research and training funds for both undergraduate and graduate nursing education; for a time, graduates whose education was supported by federal funds formed the largest cadre of master's-degree-prepared nurses in the United States. Their work and achievements in the field of psychiatric nursing are still acknowledged as having contributed enormously to the advances in psychiatric care that occurred during this period.

In 1963, expansion of the federal government's Professional Nurse Training Program, administered through the Division of Nursing of the Department of Health, Education and Welfare (DHEW), to include CNS education added a major impetus for the development of more master's degree programs to prepare CNSs in all major specialties. By 1984, there were 129 accredited master's degree programs preparing CNSs.[2] Although nurse anesthetists were the earliest of specialized nurses, CNSs became, during the 1960s and 1970s, the single largest group of nurse experts.

Today, over 58,000 CNSs provide primary, secondary, and tertiary care in all settings—hospitals, nursing homes, health departments, home care, community clinics, and solo or group practices with physicians and other health-care professionals. Psychiatric CNSs provide diagnostic and treatment services for children, adolescents, and adults, with many practicing autonomously either in their own offices or in collaboration with psychiatrists.

DEFINITION

CNSs are registered nurses (RNs) educated in master's-degree programs that prepare them to sit for the American Nurses Credentialing Center (ANCC) examination in the following areas of specialization: medical–surgical, maternal–child, psychiatric–mental health, community health, gerontology, cardiac rehabilitation, trauma, perinatal, and diabetes. A CNS, therefore, practices in one specialty area.[3]

RESPONSIBILITIES

Although each CNS practices in a chosen specialty, the responsibilities involved are common to all specialties. Thus, there are common core functions for every CNS. Georgopoulos and Christman[1] list the core functions as follows:

    1. Makes assessments of the nursing needs of patients; formulates nursing care plans, using not only nursing knowledge,

but also knowledge from the medical, biological, and social sciences; writes nursing orders, as appropriate, for the implementation of nursing plans; and generally directs the provision of care in the patient unit.

2. Makes patient assignments to the nursing staff of the unit, based on the competence of individual staff members and the nursing needs of patients; gives direct patient care as needed and appropriate.

3. Sets, evaluates, and re-evaluates standards of clinical nursing practice for the unit; communicates these standards to the nursing personnel on the unit; and, over time, changes standards as necessary.

4. Anticipates the consequences of particular clinical practices, and plans nursing care activities so as to minimize unanticipated consequences.

5. Communicates and interprets nursing assessments of patients to the medical staff and other relevant personnel; articulates nursing care designs with medical care plans and with patient service that may be rendered by other professionals; and facilitates the implementation of patient care plans.

6. Utilizes and coordinates the varied resources and facilities of the unit so as to attain and maintain high levels of nursing performance and nursing care.

7. Keeps clinical nursing records as a guide to patient care, and encourages staff members to contribute data relevant to nursing care plans, progress notes, and nursing consultation records.

8. Utilizes consultation from others, as needed.

9. Makes appropriate use of available administrative and organizational channels to facilitate, support, and maintain high levels of nursing performance.

10. Utilizes teaching and other opportunities to improve the clinical competencies of the nursing staff of the unit; communicates and interprets recent innovations and research findings to the staff; translates relevant scientific knowledge into nursing practice.

11. Introduces nursing practice innovations; refines nursing techniques and procedures; conceptualizes new formats of nursing practice; modifies particular nursing practices as appropriate.

12. Investigates specific problems of nursing practice, as appropriate, and uses the results to improve nursing performance and patient care; writes up the results of such investigations for publication.

13. Teaches patients so that they may gain better understanding of their health needs.
14. Maintains an effective communication network on the unit.
15. Attempts to maintain an environment of nursing practice that stimulates and reinforces the clinical experience of nursing students on the unit.

EDUCATION CERTIFICATION

Most master's programs can be completed in three or four semesters, with one or two summers included and considered as semesters. Many master's programs provide advanced professional tracks leading to either clinical specialist or nurse practitioner (usually in primary care).

Admission Requirements

The usual admission requirements to master's-degree programs include the following:

1. Baccalaureate degree in Nursing from a National League for Nursing-accredited school.
2. Minimum undergraduate grade point average of 3.0 on a 4.0 scale.
3. Graduate Record Examination (GRE) or Miller Analogies Test (MAT) taken within five years of application.
4. Completion of the Graduate School Admissions Application.
5. Completion of a Professional Goals Statement.
6. Three letters of recommendation—two from academic institutions.
7. Official transcripts from every undergraduate and graduate institution attended.
8. Satisfactory completion of an introductory three-credit course in statistical methods.
9. Registered nurse license.
10. One year of professional nursing practice in appropriate clinical area.
11. Preadmission interview.
12. Test of English as a Foreign Language (TOEFL) score of 580 or higher for students who are not native speakers of English.

If admitted, students must provide evidence of health insurance coverage and liability insurance coverage (these requirements vary with schools).

Curriculum

In most schools of nursing, all master's degree students are required to take a particular number of required core courses, such as:

- Theoretical Foundations of Nursing
- Principles of Biostatistics
- Research Methods
- Clinical Ethics: Theory and Practice
- Advanced Health Assessment
- Health Care Systems
- Health Promotion and Disease Prevention

Additional requirements are based on the program in which the student enrolls; for example, students in advanced practice nursing programs are usually required to take courses in advanced pharmacology and advanced pathophysiology.

Clinical experiences and other courses are arranged according to clinical specialty. The total number of credits required varies by program, but usually ranges from 36 to 48 credits.

Certification of CNSs

The ANCC offers certification examinations for clinical nurse specialists in five specialty areas: medical–surgical nursing, gerontological nursing, community health nursing, home health nursing, psychiatric and mental health nursing.

SPECIALTIES

Clinical Specialist in Medical–Surgical Nursing

Master's-degree-prepared CNSs in medical–surgical nursing care for patients who have known or predicted physiological alterations. CNSs demonstrate an in-depth understanding of complex medical–surgical problems and interventions to manage and improve patient care. Guided by theory and research, the CNS considers all influences on health status and the related social and behavioral problems arising because of the patient's condition. CNSs are engaged in education, expert clinical practice, consultation, research, and administration. Practice sites include primary, acute, secondary, home care, and long-term nursing care facilities.

Eligibility requirements to take the ANCC certification examination are:

1. An active RN license in the United States or its territories.
2. A master's degree in nursing.
3. Demonstration of current direct patient care in medical-surgical nursing an average of 4 hours (or more) per week.
4. Demonstration of practice (with an active U.S. RN license) for a minimum of 12 months following completion of the master's degree.
5. A minimum of 800 hours of direct patient care within the past 24 months *or* full-time employment as a consultant, researcher, administrator, or educator for two of the past three years *and* direct medical-surgical nursing care of patients for a minimum of 400 hours during this time.

Topic areas included in the certification examination are clinical practice, consultation, management, education, research, and issues and trends.

Clinical Specialist in Gerontological Nursing

CNSs in gerontological nursing are experts in providing, directing, and influencing the care of older adults and their families and caregivers in a variety of settings. CNSs demonstrate an in-depth understanding of the dynamics of aging and the interventions necessary for health promotion and management of health problems. CNSs provide comprehensive gerontological nursing services independently or collaboratively with a multidisciplinary team. Through theory and research, CNSs advance the health care of older persons, the role of the gerontological CNS, and are engaged in practice, case management, education, consultation, research, and administration.

Eligibility requirements for the gerontological CNS are the same as the requirements for the medical–surgical specialty: licensure as an RN, master's degree in gerontological nursing, practice time and hours. In 1998, the educational requirement will be a master's degree in gerontological nursing *or* a master's degree in nursing with specialization in gerontological nursing.

The topic areas included in the examination are practice, education, consultation, research, and administration.

Clinical Specialist in Community Health Nursing

The master's-degree-prepared community health nurse CNS performs all functions of the community health generalist, possesses substantial clinical experience in the assessment of the health of a community, and has proficiency in planning, implementing, and evaluating population-focused programs. The skills of this specialist are based on knowledge of epidemiology, demography, biometrics, environmental health, community structure and organization, community development, management, program evaluation, and policy development. The CNS in community health nursing engages in research and theory application relevant to community practice and health policy development. Although there are graduate-prepared nurses whose area of expertise is the care of a particular segment of the community, the practice of the community health nurse CNS emphasizes the use of skills to promote the health of an entire community.
Eligibility requirements are:

1. Master's degree in nursing with a specialization in community/public health nursing practice *or* master's degree in nursing *or* baccalaureate degree in nursing *and* a master's or higher degree in public health.
2. Effective in 1998, master's or higher degree in nursing, with a specialization in community or public health nursing *or* baccalaureate or higher degree in nursing *and* a master's degree in public health with a specialization in community/public health nursing.

The topic areas included in the examination are public health sciences, community assessment process, program administration, trends and issues, theory, research, and health-care delivery system.

Clinical Specialist in Home Health Nursing

Home health nursing involves the practice of caring for a client with a health deficit at the client's place of residence or other appropriate community site. The graduate-prepared CNS in home health nursing practice can and may be asked to perform all the functions of a generalist. In addition, this CNS possesses substantial clinical experience with all types of clients—individuals, families, and groups. The home health CNS has expertise in the process of case management, consultation, collaboration, and the education of clients, staff, and other health professionals. In addition, the home health CNS has proficiency in planning, implementing, and evaluating programs, resources, services, and research for health-care delivery to clients who have complex problems.

Eligibility requirements are:

1. An active RN license in the United States or its territories
2. A master's or higher degree in nursing
3. Demonstration of practice as a licensed RN in home health nursing for a minimum of 1000 hours within the past 24 months, following conferral of the master's degree in nursing or graduation from a master's degree in nursing program for CNS in home health (up to 50% of the clinical practice within the graduate program may be applied toward the completion of the 1000-hour practice requirement)
4. Demonstration of current direct patient care or clinical management in home health nursing for at least an *average* of 8 hours a week.

Topic areas included in the examination are practice, education, consultation, research, administration, and issues and trends. The examination also requires a completed application and Rapid Response Form, answers to questions in Section Q of the Nursing Practice Questionnaire, and a copy of a transcript or diploma verifying conferral of master's degree in nursing.

Clinical Specialist in Adult or Child/Adolescent Psychiatric and Mental Health Nursing

CNSs in psychiatric and mental health nursing possess a high degree of proficiency in therapeutic and interpersonal skills. These specialists influence and modify attitudes and behaviors of patients, and assume responsibility for the advancement of nursing theory and therapy. Roles of the psychiatric and mental health CNS include teaching, research, consultation, supervision, case management, and administration.

The eligibility criteria required to take the examination are licensure, master's degree in psychiatric and mental health nursing, practice an average of 4 hours per week, current involvement in clinical consultation or clinical supervision, and experience in at least two different treatment modalities. Effective in 1996, 12 of the 24 academic credits required in psychiatric and mental health theory must be in psychiatric mental health *nursing* theory.

Topic areas included in the examination are practice theories, psychopathology, treatment modalities, lifestyle and environment, trends and issues, education, and consultation and research.

SUMMARY

The core functions of the CNS clearly indicate that the CNS role was initially a nursing role. Because the CNS has a high level of education and expert knowledge of particular areas of nursing, the nursing staff is able to have a resource person and can attain a high level of performance in providing care to patients. From the 1960s through the 1980s, the effectiveness of CNSs, shown by outcomes of care and patient and staff satisfaction was evident in many hospitals.[1]

Today, because of managed care and hospitals' reengineering resulting in downsizing and elimination of staff, CNSs may be in more demand in settings other than acute care, for example, in home health care, health departments, community clinics, and private or group practices. CNSs with experience and expertise are particularly in demand to care for critically ill patients in the home.

The need for expert nurse clinicians is as great as ever, but the means to support both CNSs and NPs are no longer available. To remain solvent, hospitals and other care facilities are scaling back and retaining only the most essential and effective staff. CNSs have a 40-year history of managing acute and long-term care needs of patients with complex problems; coordinating the discharge-planning process through assessment of a family's home care capabilities, support, and physical environment; developing plans for transitional care; improving outcomes through follow-up and monitoring; and coordinating care as case managers.

REFERENCES

1. Georgopoulos S, Christman, L. Effects of clinical nursing specialization: A controlled organizational experiment. *Studies in Health and Human Services,* Vol. 14. Lewiston, NY: The Edwin Mellen Press, 1990.
2. American Nurses' Association. *Information in the Database.* Washington, DC: American Nurses' Association, 1996.
3. American Nurses Credentialing Center. *1996 Certification Catalog.* Washington, DC: American Nurses Credentialing Center, 1996.

BIBLIOGRAPHY

Hamric AB, Spross JA. *The Clinical Nurse Specialist in Theory and Practice.* Philadel-
     phia: Saunders, 1989.
Peplau HE. Specialization in professional nursing. *Nurs Sci,* 3(8):268–287, 1965.
Reiter F. The nurse-clinician. *Am J Nurs,* 66(2):274–280, 1966.

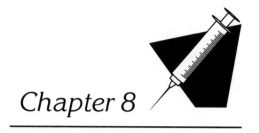

Chapter 8

Certified Registered
Nurse Anesthetists

A Certified Registered Nurse Anesthetist (CRNA) practices primarily in hospital operating rooms in all aspects of anesthesia care, which includes complete examination and assessment of the patient the evening before the procedure; determination of the patient's physical and psychological status with respect to the type of anesthesia to be given; selection and ordering of appropriate preoperative medications; induction of anesthesia at the start of the procedure; monitoring the patient continuously throughout the procedure; and managing the patient's recovery from anesthesia in the postoperative period. Although CRNAs are nurses, not physicians, their theoretical knowledge base and clinical skills in all aspects of patient care regarding anesthesia are considered to be equivalent to the skills of physicians who are trained to be anesthesiologists, since CRNAs are able to care for patients undergoing all types of surgical procedures, from simple to the most complex. Supervision by anesthesiologists of CRNAs' practice is not a legal requirement in any state. Other sites in which CRNAs practice include physicians' offices, clinics, dentists' offices, and anywhere that patients may require administration of anesthesia. CRNA educational programs are becoming master's-degree programs in university settings to educate nurse anesthetists at the graduate level. This trend has been in process only since the late 1980s, but many CRNAs held bachelor's or master's degrees in nursing before becoming CRNAs; they therefore had advanced preparation in nursing before entering the field of anesthesia.

HISTORY

Nurses were the first professional group to provide anesthesia services in the United States. Established in the late 1800s as the first clinical nursing specialty, CRNA training developed in response to the growing need surgeons had for specially trained anesthetists. In 1877, Sister Mary Bernard of St. Vincent's Hospital in Erie, Pennsylvania, became the first identified nurse anesthetist. A few years later, two German religious sisters, Aldonza Elrich and Vanossa Woenke of the Third Order of the Hospital Sisters of St. Francis, had been trained by surgeons to administer anesthesia. They emigrated to the United States, established a religious community in Illinois, and began to practice anesthesia in nearby hospitals.

St. Mary's Hospital (now the Mayo Clinic) in Rochester, Minnesota, was established by Dr. William Worrell Mayo in 1889. Dr. Mayo, along with Alice Magaw, whom he identified as the "mother of anesthesia," were instrumental in setting up a showcase of professional excellence in surgery and anesthesia. Both physicians and nurses came to observe and learn anesthesia techniques from this team. Alice Magaw documented the anesthesia practice outcomes at St. Mary's Hospital and reported them in various medical journals between 1899 and 1906. During this period, the idea of formalizing the education of nurses as anesthetists became operationalized in the manual of education that included both theoretic and clinical experiences for RNs wishing to become anesthetists.

World War I greatly increased the demand for anesthetists and resulted in the escalation of the number of nurses being prepared in this specialty. Experienced CRNAs trained both physicians and nurses to provide anesthesia services at home and abroad to meet the demand for anesthetists in the field hospitals close to the battlefields. CRNAs who had trained in the United States and who were attached to field hospitals trained physicians and nurses from allied countries whenever possible.

CRNAs have been the principal anesthesia providers in combat areas in every war the United States has been engaged in since World War I. CRNAs have received medals and accolades for their dedication, commitment, and competence. In World War II, the ratio of CRNAs to physician anesthesiologists was 17 to 1. In Vietnam, the ratio was about 3 to 1. During the Panama strike in 1994, only CRNAs were sent with the fighting forces. Several CRNAs have suffered combat wounds during wartime service; two who were killed in Vietnam have their names engraved on the Vietnam Memorial Wall in Washington, DC. Many CRNAs received both U.S. and foreign decorations and medals for their contributions during World War I, World War II, the Korean War, the Vietnam War, and the brief Persian Gulf War.

CRNAs have been pioneers in anesthesia for specialty surgery, particularly that related to lung and open heart surgery. Kitty Rolands was the nurse anesthetist in attendance at the world's first open heart procedure in which a heart-lung machine (oxygenator) was used successfully for the first time. The operation to correct an atrial septal defect took place on May 6, 1953, at Philadelphia's Jefferson Hospital, with Dr. John Heysham Gibbon, Jr., the developer of the oxygenator, as the surgeon.[1]

Although some physicians devoted their practices to anesthesia and made significant contributions during World War I, the formalization of physician education in anesthesia did not occur until after World War II. At the outbreak of World War II, only seven anesthesiology residencies, consisting of about one year of specialty training, existed for physicians.

AMERICAN ASSOCIATION OF NURSE ANESTHETISTS

Founded in 1931, the American Association of Nurse Anesthetists (AANA) is the national professional association that represents more than 27,000 CRNAs. The primary goal of the AANA has been the development of educational and practice standards for CRNAs. The AANA implemented a certification process for nurse anesthetists in 1945 and instituted mandatory recertification in 1978. It established a mechanism for accreditation of nurse anesthesia education programs in 1952, which has been recognized by the U.S. Department of Education since 1955. Thus, the AANA was a leader in forming multidisciplinary councils with public representation to fulfill the profession's autonomous credentialing functions.

The AANA, in collaboration with its credentialing councils, continues to update educational and practice standards; its accreditation, certification, and recertification processes; and develops position statements and guidelines. The credentialing processes are broadly recognized by public and private agencies. Ninety-six percent of CRNAs are AANA members, which represents the highest membership in any professional organization within nursing.

SCOPE OF PRACTICE

The practice of anesthesia is a recognized specialty in both nursing and medicine. *Anesthesiology* is the art and science of rendering a patient insensible to pain through the administration of anesthetic agents and related drugs and procedures. Anesthesia and anesthesia-related care represents those services that anesthesia professionals provide on request, assignment, and referral by the patient's physician or other health-care provider authorized by law, most often to facilitate diagnostic, therapeutic, and surgical procedures. In other instances, the referral or request for consultation or assistance may be for the management of pain associated with obstetrical labor and delivery, management of acute and chronic ventilatory problems, or the management of acute and chronic pain through the performance of selected diagnostic and therapeutic blocks or other forms of pain management. CRNAs practice according to their expertise, state statutes and regulations, and institutional policy.

CRNA scope of practice includes, but is not limited to, the following:

1. Performing and documenting a preanesthetic assessment and evaluation of the patient, including requesting consultations and diagnostic studies; selecting, obtaining, ordering, and administering pre-anesthetic medications and fluids; and obtaining informed consent for anesthesia.
2. Developing and implementing an anesthetic plan.
3. Initiating the anesthetic technique, which may include general, regional, local, and sedation.
4. Selecting, applying, and inserting appropriate noninvasive and invasive monitoring modalities for continuous evaluation of the patient's physical status.
5. Selecting, obtaining, and administering the anesthetics, adjuvant and accessory drugs, and fluids necessary to manage the anesthetic.
6. Managing a patient's airway and pulmonary status using current practice modalities.
7. Managing emergence and recovery from anesthesia by selecting, obtaining, ordering, and administering fluids, medications, and ventilatory support.
8. Discharging the patient from a postanesthesia care area and providing postanesthesia follow-up evaluation and care.
9. Implementing acute and chronic pain management modalities.
10. Responding to emergency situations by providing airway management, administration of emergency fluids and drugs, and using basic or advanced cardiac life support techniques.

Additional nurse anesthesia responsibilities that are within the expertise of the individual CRNA include:

1. *Administration/management*—scheduling; material and supply management; supervision of staff, students, or ancillary personnel; development of policies and procedures; fiscal management; performance evaluations; and preventive maintenance, billing, and data management.

2. *Quality assessment*—data collection, reporting mechanism, trending, compliance, committee meetings, departmental review, problem-focused studies, problem solving, interventions, documents, and process oversight.
3. *Educational*—clinical and didactic teaching, BCLS/ACLS instruction, inservice commitment, EMT training, supervision of residents, and facility continuing education.
4. *Research*—conducting and participating in departmental, hospital-wide, and university-sponsored research projects.
5. *Committee appointments*—assignment to committees, committee responsibilities, and coordination of committee activities.
6. *Interdepartmental liaison*—interface with other departments such as nursing, surgery, obstetrics, postanesthesia care units (PACU), outpatient surgery, admissions, administration, laboratory, pharmacy, and so on.
7. *Clinical/administrative oversight of other departments*—respiratory therapy, PACU, operating room, surgical intensive care unit (SICU), pain clinics, and so on.

The functions listed here are a summary of CRNA clinical practice and are not intended to be all-inclusive. A more specific list of CRNA functions and practice parameters is detailed in the *Guidelines for Granting Clinical Privileges to Certified Registered Nurse Anesthetists.*[3]

CRNAs strive for professional excellence by demonstrating competence and commitment to the clinical, educational, consultative, research, and administrative practice in the specialty of anesthesia. CRNAs should actively participate in the development of departmental policies and guidelines, performance appraisals, peer reviews, clinical and administrative conferences, and serve on health-care facility committees. In addition to these activities, CRNAs should assume a leadership role in the evaluation of the quality of anesthesia care provided throughout the facility and the community.

STANDARDS OF PRACTICE

A characteristic of any profession is its responsibility to the public to develop a code of ethics and practice standards by which the quality of practice rendered by its members can be assessed. Standards based on sound philosophy, theory, science, principles, and a code of ethics continually upgrade clinical practice.

The practice standards developed by the AANA are intended to assist the CRNA in providing consistent, safe anesthesia care. The standards are descriptive, thus providing a basis for evaluating the practice and reflecting the rights of patients receiving anesthesia care. The AANA recognizes that it may not be possible for the CRNA to comply with each standard in particular extraordinary or emergency situations. However, it is expected that CRNAs assess each situation and use professional judgment in deciding the appropriate anesthetic plan to ensure a safe anesthetic course for the patient.

Practice standards strongly encourage high-quality patient care, but they cannot ensure specific patient outcomes, which rest on multiple factors. The intent of practice standards is to:

1. Assist the profession by evaluating the quality of care provided by its practitioners.
2. Provide a common base for practitioners to use in coordinating care and unifying efforts in promoting quality practice.
3. Assist the public in understanding what to expect from the practitioners.
4. Support and preserve the basic rights of the patient.

The AANA Code of Ethics is reprinted in Appendix D, and the practice standards of the AANA are reprinted in Appendix E.

EDUCATION/CERTIFICATION

The most significant difference between CRNAs and anesthesiologists (physicians) is that, prior to entering anesthesia education, anesthesiologists receive medical education and CRNAs receive nursing education. However, the theory and practical educational aspects of administering anesthesia are similar for both groups; both are prepared to provide the full range of anesthesia and related services.

As of November 1995, there were 90 accredited CRNA education programs in the United States, of which 97% offer a master's degree. The other 3% of programs are modifying their curriculums to offer the master's degree beginning in 1998. Some CRNA programs are offering both master's degrees and clinical nursing doctoral degrees as an option for nurses pursuing graduate preparation. Other programs are considering the clinical nursing doctorate as the entry-level requirement for nurse anesthetists.[4]

Admission Requirements

An individual applying to a CRNA education program must, in general, meet these criteria:

- Hold a bachelor of science in nursing (BSN), or other appropriate baccalaureate degree.
- Be licensed as a registered nurse (RN) in at least one state.
- Have a minimum of one year of critical care nursing experience.

Individual institutions may vary in additional requirements for admission to nurse anesthesia programs. Examples of additional requirements include:

- Have taken an undergraduate statistics course.
- Have taken an undergraduate course in physical assessment (all body systems).
- Have three letters of reference/recommendation in the application packet.
- Arrange an interview with a faculty member from the program prior to being considered for admission to the graduate program.

Curriculum

In general, CRNA education programs consist of 24 to 36 months of full-time graduate work, which includes both classroom (theory) and clinical experience. The undergraduate curriculum requirements typically include coursework and appropriate laboratory experience in anatomy, physiology, and pathophysiology; biochemistry and physics related to anesthesia; advanced pharmacology; principles of anesthesia practice; research methodology and statistical analysis; and research or other scholarly endeavors.

The master's degree clinical curriculum provides experiences with a variety of anesthesia techniques and procedures for all types of surgery and obstetrics. All CRNA master's degree programs are rigorous. The following list of course requirements for one specific school of nursing are presented as an example. In this specific school, the master's degree is conferred on completion of 90 quarter hours (about 60 semester hours) of coursework and clinical practice. The program requires two years plus one summer of full-time study. Required courses include:

Dimensions of Contemporary Health Care (4 qhrs)

Conceptual Matrix for Nursing: Health and Illness (2 qhrs)

Conceptual Matrix for Nursing: Human Behavior and Nursing (2 qhrs)

Conceptual Matrix for Nursing: Nursing Concepts and Theories (2 qhrs)

Research Design and Inference I (4 qhrs)

Research Seminar (thesis–8 qhrs; research project—4 qhrs plus an elective course, 4 qhrs)

Physiological Applications in Nurse Anesthesia I (3 qhrs)

Physiological Applications in Nurse Anesthesia II (3 qhrs)

Physiological Applications in Nurse Anesthesia III (4 qhrs)

Physiological Applications in Nurse Anesthesia IV (3 qhrs)

Physiological Applications in Nurse Anesthesia V (2 qhrs)

Theoretical Principles of Anesthetic Management I (3 qhrs)

Theoretical Principles of Anesthetic Management II (4 qhrs)

Theoretical Principles of Anesthetic Management III (4 qhrs)

Anesthesia Clinical Lab/Practice (1 qhr)

Nurse Anesthesia Clinical Practice II (2 qhrs)

Nurse Anesthesia Clinical Practice III (2 qhrs)

Nurse Anesthesia Clinical Practice IV (2 qhrs)

Nurse Anesthesia Clinical Practice V (2 qhrs)

Advanced Pharmacology (4 qhrs)

Adjunctive Anesthetic Pharmacology (2 qhrs)

Anesthetic Pharmacology (3 qhrs)

Analysis/Synthesis of Anesthetic Concepts I (2 qhrs)

Analysis/Synthesis of Anesthetic Concepts II (3 qhrs)

Analysis/Synthesis of Anesthetic Concepts III (3 qhrs)

Advanced Nursing in Perioperative Care (3 qhrs)

Advanced Nursing in Respiratory Care (2 qhrs)

Professional Dimensions in Nurse Anesthesia I (2 qhrs)

Professional Dimensions in Nurse Anesthesia II (3 qhrs)

Nurse Anesthesia Practice Practicum (4 qhrs, 240 clinical hrs)

Graduation requirements in this particular school of nursing include meeting those of the university *plus* the following for students in the CRNA program:

- At least 450 contact hours of didactic coursework
- At least 450 anesthetic cases with 800 hours of actual anesthesia administration
- Advanced Cardiorespiratory Life Support (ACLS) certification

- Satisfactory monthly or bimonthly clinical evaluations
- Completion of a written exit evaluation of all components of the program
- An exit interview by the Nurse Anesthesia Evaluation Committee of the School of Nursing.

Accreditation of Nurse Anesthesia Education Programs

Since 1975, the AANA Council on Accreditation of Nurse Anesthesia Educational Programs has been the body responsible for promulgating, publishing, and assessing compliance of programs with the *Scope and Standards for Programs of Nurse Anesthesia*.[2] Prior to 1975, the AANA was the recognized accrediting body of CRNA programs, but in 1975, the Department of Health, Education, and Welfare required that the accrediting body become a separate entity to ensure greater objectivity and validity in the accreditation process. The AANA Council on Accreditation (COA) was formed at that time. COA comprises multidisciplinary membership and is recognized by the Department of Education and the Commission on Recognition of Post-Secondary Accreditation (CORPA) as the sole accrediting authority for CRNA programs. Recognition by these bodies is important not only for validating the quality of the educational programs but also because such recognition ensures eligibility for federal grant funds and federal student financial assistance.

COA requires that each program undergo a systematic self-study and onsite evaluation at least every six years to document that every program is in compliance with the standards of COA regarding the overall excellence of the didactic and clinical portions of the curriculum, clinical practicum experiences, and faculty qualifications and expertise for supervising student experiences. Annually, COA publishes a list of accredited CRNA educational programs.

Certification of Nurse Anesthetists

The primary purpose of certification is to protect and serve the public by assuming that individuals who are credentialed have met predetermined qualifications or standards for providing nurse anesthesia services.

At the first meeting of the National Association of Nurse Anesthetists (NANA) in 1933, planning began for the development of a national certification examination. Certification provides employers of nurse anesthetists—physicians and hospitals—official documentation of the knowledge level and minimal clinical competencies of individual CRNAs.

The certification process was introduced by the AANA in 1945. In 1975, the AANA recognized the Council on Certification of Nurse Anesthetists (CCNA) as an autonomous entity having the functions to certify, protect, and benefit the public by documenting the qualifications and competence of CRNAs.

Credentialing is recognized as a process different from licensure. State licensure provides the legal credential for the practice of professional nursing. Certification shows compliance with professional standards of practice and minimal competencies of the individual to practice within the scope indicated by the profession. The certification credential for CRNAs has been continually recognized in proceedings involving malpractice litigation, selected state nurse practice acts, and state and federal regulations.

To take the national certification examination an applicant must (1) hold a current, valid state RN license; (2) be a graduate of a COA-accredited CRNA education program; (3) submit a completed application form; (4) provide a notarized transcript from the CRNA program to document the applicant's academic and clinical experiences; (5) have no mental or physical conditions that may interfere with practice; (6) have no convictions of a felony nor be under indictment; and (7) not have been subject to any documented allegations of misconduct, incompetent practice, or unethical behavior.

The CCNA maintains responsibility for the examination content, the test specifications, and an item bank of test questions; approves an individual's application to take the examination; and determines the passing score.

Recertification of Nurse Anesthetists

In 1976, members of the AANA amended the bylaws to make continuing education (CE) mandatory for all CRNAs. The AANA recognized the importance of continually demonstrating professional excellence among its members and, in 1978, the Council on Recertification became the fourth autonomous body within the organization. The purpose of recertification is to ensure that all nurse anesthetists continue to maintain their level of scientific and technical knowledge and skills. Every two years, CRNAs must renew their certification, which requires that candidates must have (1) initial certification; (2) a current RN license with no restrictions; (3) completion of 40 hours of continuing education in a two-year period; (4) substantial engagement in the practice of anesthesia; (5) no mental or physical conditions that may interfere with practice; (6) no convictions of a felony nor be under indictment; and (7) not been subject to any documented allegations of misconduct, incompetent practice, or unethical behavior.

Licensing and Liability

Some state licensing laws and regulations require CRNAs to practice under the supervision or direction of a surgeon, dentist, podiatrist, or other specialist. However, neither state licensing statutes nor the Joint Commission on Accreditation of Health Care Organizations (JCAHO) requires CRNAs to be supervised by anesthesiologists.

In addition, liability is the same whether surgeons work with CRNAs or with anesthesiologists. Whether a surgeon is held liable for events that may occur during a specific surgical case depends on the facts related to the case, not to the individual administering anesthesia. Since 1984, St. Paul Fire and Marine Insurance Company has been the underwriter for the AANA Professional Liability Insurance Program; it is the largest medical malpractice underwriter in the United States and bases its annual professional liability insurance premium for CRNAs on previous claim losses. For the past three years, the annual premium rate has dropped an average of 6% because of the low number of claim losses incurred by CRNAs.

REFERENCES

1. Romaine-Davis A. *John Gibbon and His Heart-Lung Machine*. Philadelphia: University of Pennsylvania Press, 1991.
2. American Association of Nurse Anesthetists. *Scope and Standards for Nurse Anesthesia Practice*. Park Ridge, IL: American Association of Nurse Anesthetists, 1996.
3. American Association of Nurse Anesthetists. *Guidelines for Granting Privileges to Certified Nurse Anesthetists*. Park Ridge, IL: American Association of Nurse Anesthetists, 1992.
4. Cordes VK, Public Relations Specialist, American Association of Nurse Anesthetists, Park Ridge, IL. Personal communication, October 1995.

BIBLIOGRAPHY

American Association of Nurse Anesthetists. *Professional and Legal Issues of Nurse Anesthesia Practice*. Park Ridge, IL: American Association of Nurse Anesthetists, 1989.

Foster SC, Jordan LM, eds. *Professional Aspects of Nurse Anesthesia Practice*. Park Ridge, IL: American Association of Nurse Anesthetists, 1994.

Gravenstein JS, Holzer, JF, eds. *Safety and Cost Containment in Anesthesia*. Stoneham, MA: Butterworth–Heinemann, 1988.

Rosenbach ML, Cromwell J. *Payment Options for Non-Physician Anesthetists Under Medicare's Prospective Payment System*. Report prepared under Health Care Financing Administration Cooperative Agreement (No. 18-C-98759/1-02). Needham, MA: Center for Health Economics Research, 1988.

Part III

Professional Issues

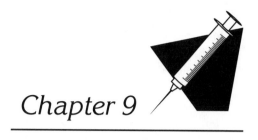

Chapter 9

Reimbursement

History
Public Sources of Reimbursement
Private Sources of Reimbursement

HISTORY

When an individual requests services and they are provided by the persons best qualified to render them, the persons rendering the services have the right to require fair compensation. Advanced practice nurses (APNs) have spent considerable time and money in acquiring knowledge and skills that enable them to provide high-quality services to patients, and APNs should be reimbursed for their expertise.

Traditionally, physician assistants (PAs), nurse practitioners (NPs), certified nurse-midwives (CNMs), clinical nurse specialists (CNSs), and certified registered nurse anesthetists (CRNAs) were employed by hospitals, physicians in group practices, or by individual private physicians. The appropriate sources were billed for the services provided by the physician and by the APN. The hospital, physician group, or private physician paid the APN. In these situations, and until only recently, APNs had little knowledge or understanding of the reimbursement system, and no education about managing the business aspect of their professional practice. Accustomed to working as paid employees, APNs simply assumed that they were being fairly compensated; most had no idea of the exact worth of their professional services. However, in the early 1980s, APNs became more aware of their rights as providers of care to request appropriate and fair reimbursement for their services, and their professional organizations began to lobby for the rights of APNs.

Reimbursement is available through several sources, both public and private. Public reimbursement comes through Medicare, Medicaid, state mandates, the Federal Employee Health Benefit Program (FEHBP), and the Civilian Health and Medical Program of Uniformed Services (CHAMPUS). Private sources of reimbursement include payment through fee-for-service and private insurance companies such as Blue Cross/Blue Shield, Mutual of Omaha, Prudential, and others.

PUBLIC SOURCES OF REIMBURSEMENT
Medicare

The Medicare program covers hospital, physicians' services, and other medical services for most persons 65 years of age or older, disabled persons entitled to social security cash benefits for at least 24 months, and most persons with end-stage renal disease. Major changes in the Medicare law through the Omnibus Budget Reconciliation Act (OBRA) of 1986 (Public Law 99-509) enabled direct reimbursement to nonphysician providers. Total Medicare benefit payments (reimbursement and other payments from Medicare trust funds) totaled $79.8 billion in 1987.

Medicare has two complementary but distinct parts: hospital insurance (HI), also called Part A, and supplementary medical insurance (SMI), called Part B. The HI program covers 90 days of inpatient hospital care in a benefit period (episode or illness) that begins with the first day of hospitalization and ends when the beneficiary has not been an inpatient in a hospital or skilled nursing facility (SNF) for 60 consecutive days. There is no limit to the number of benefit periods an individual may use. The program also provides a nonrenewable (lifetime) reserve of 60 days if a beneficiary exhausts the 90 days available in a benefit period.

In addition to inpatient hospital care, the HI program covers up to 100 posthospital days in an SNF if the beneficiary is certified by a physician to require such care. The HI program also covers home health agency visits.

About 95% of the nation's aged are enrolled in the HI program. On July 1, 1966, when Medicare became operational, 19.1 million older persons were enrolled. By July 1, 1986, the number of enrollees had increased to 31.7 million, which included 3.0 million disabled persons. Medicare coverage of the disabled began on July 1, 1973.

Nearly everyone covered by HI voluntarily enrolls in SMI. Unlike HI, SMI requires a monthly premium payment, which increased from $24.80 per month in 1988 to $27.90 in 1989. Under buy-in agreements, most state Medicaid programs pay the premiums for persons who qualify for both Medicaid and Medicare benefits. The SMI program provides payments for physicians and for related services and supplies ordered by physicians. SMI also covers outpatient hospital services, rural health clinic visits, and home health visits.

Several health-care services, such as routine eye examinations and preventive services, are widely used by older persons but are not covered by Medicare. Drugs and certain dental procedures are covered only if provided during an authorized hospital inpatient stay. Neither intermediate nor long-term nursing care is covered by Medicare.

Both the HI and SMI programs require beneficiary cost sharing. Under HI, the patient is required to pay an inpatient hospital deductible for each benefit period. The Secretary of Health and Human Services set the annual HI deductible in 1988 at $540, based on a formula specified by law. The co-insurance amount is based on percentages of the inpatient hospital deductible. Co-insurance equal to one-fourth the hospital deductible is required from day 61 through day 90 of inpatient hospital care. An amount equal to one-eighth the deductible is required from day 21 through day 100 of SNF care. An amount equal to one-half the deductible is required for the 60 lifetime reserve days for inpatient hospital care. The patient is also liable for the cost of replacement of the first three pints of blood used in a benefit period. Under SMI, in addition to paying a monthly premium, the beneficiary must pay a $75 deductible each year.

Physicians can accept or reject assignment. Acceptance of assignment means that participating physicians agree to accept as full payment the amount Medicare allows for the service. The program reimburses 80% of allowed (reasonable) charges directly to the physician. Beneficiaries are liable for the remaining 20% of allowed charges (co-insurance). Nonparticipating physicians do not agree to accept assignment. On unassigned claims, the beneficiary is responsible for the difference between the physician's charges and the allowed charge and for the 20% co-insurance. The Medicaid program assumes cost sharing for Medicaid enrollees covered under buy-in agreements. As of December 1987, only three Medicaid jurisdictions did not have a buy-in program.

Medicare benefits and administrative expenses are paid from two separate trust funds. The HI trust fund is financed primarily through a tax on current earnings from employment covered by the Social Security Act. The SMI trust fund is financed through premiums paid by or on behalf of persons enrolled in the program and from general revenues of the federal government.

Medicare Reimbursement Incident to Physicians' Services

Since the beginning of Medicare, the services delivered by a physician's employee and the supplies furnished have been considered "incident to" the physician's service; they have either been included in a physician's bill or delivered without charge. Under this rule, the services delivered by RNs, NPs, CNSs, and CRNAs who are employees of the physician, are frequently charged to Medicare using the physician's provider number. Payment is received at the full rate, as though the physician had delivered the service.

Except in the case of rural health clinic services and the services of health maintenance organizations (HMOs) and other competitive medical plans, services and supplies rendered in private-practice settings can be considered incident to a physician's professional services only if there is direct personal supervision by the physician. The rule applies to employees of the practice who work under the physician's direct supervision: nurses, nonphysician anesthetists, psychologists, technicians, therapists, and others. *Direct personal supervision* means that the physician must be present in the office suite and immediately available to provide assistance and direction throughout the time the employee is performing services.[1]

Medicaid

Medicaid is supported by both federal and state funds. It is a state-administered assistance program providing medical care for qualifying low-income individuals and families. Medicaid accounted for $41 billion in federal and state expenditures for medical services in 1986.

Certain groups must be covered by state Medicaid programs. The mandatory groups generally fit two broad categories. The first consists of low-income families with dependent children. Historically, this group comprised only families receiving cash assistance through the Aid to Families with Dependent Children (AFDC) program, but recent legislation has expanded Medicaid eligibility in this area to include other low-income families. The second category consists of low-income aged and disabled persons. Generally, this group includes individuals receiving cash assistance through the Social Security Supplemental Security Income (SSI) program and certain SSI-related groups. States may also cover other groups, including groups related to the mandatory coverage groups such as medically needy persons. The *medically needy* are individuals whose incomes or resources are above the levels generally required for eligibility but who have incurred large medical expenses.

Title XIX of the Social Security Act requires that every state Medicaid program offer certain basic services: inpatient hospital services, outpatient hospital services, laboratory and x-ray services, SNF services for individuals 21 years of age or older, home health services for individuals eligible for

SNF services, physicians' services, family planning services, rural health clinic services, nurse-midwife services, and early and periodic screening, diagnosis, and treatment services for individuals under 21 years of age. States may also elect to provide a number of other services, including prescription drugs, eyeglasses, private-duty nursing, intermediate-care facility services, inpatient psychiatric care for the aged and for persons under 21 years old, physical therapy, and dental care.

Medicaid is a *vendor payment* program: payments are made directly to providers of service for care rendered to eligible individuals. Providers who choose to participate in the program must accept the Medicaid reimbursement levels as full payment. States have wide latitude in choosing methods of provider reimbursement.

As mentioned, Medicaid is financed jointly with state and federal funds. Federal contributions vary according to each state's per capita income; federal contributions currently range from 50% to 80% of program medical expenditures. Administrative costs are financed at other rates.

By the end of 1987, most state Medicaid programs had buy-in agreements with Medicare. Under these agreements, Medicaid paid the Part B Medicare premiums and cost sharing for persons covered by both programs. Medicare, in turn, paid for the costs of Medicare-covered services for the dually enrolled population. The Medicare Catastrophic Coverage Act of 1988 (Public Law 100-234) made Medicaid buy-in of Medicare coverage mandatory for qualified Medicare beneficiaries (QMBs) as of January 1, 1989. QMBs are elderly and disabled persons whose incomes are at or below specified percentages of the federal poverty level. This provision was retained despite subsequent repeal of major portions of the legislation.

States administer their Medicaid programs within broad federal requirements and guidelines. The requirements allow states considerable discretion in determining income and other resource criteria for eligibility, covered benefits, and provider payment mechanisms. Therefore, Medicaid programs vary considerably from state to state.

Medicare and Medicaid were administered by separate agencies in the Department of Health, Education and Welfare from 1965 to 1977. In 1977, the agencies were merged into the Health Care Financing Administration (HCFA) within the Department of Health and Human Services. Under that structure, the operation of Medicare and Medicaid was combined, with each newly created bureau or office dealing with a specific aspect of both programs. An intermediate level of associate administrators was added in 1981. The four associate administrators and the four staff offices report to the Administrator and the Deputy Administrator.

Medicaid Reimbursement

According to the Medicaid implementing instructions entitled *State Medicaid Manual Part 4—Services, August 1990,* services rendered by certified family nurse practitioners (CFNPs) and certified pediatric nurse practitioners (CPNPs) are covered by state Medicaid agencies according to individual state nurse practice acts regarding the scope of practice allowed by law for the NPs and regardless of whether the NPs were supervised by or associated with a physician or other health-care provider. Medicaid agencies are directed to offer direct payment to these NPs as an option.

Almost all states allow APNs to be directly reimbursed for providing care to Medicaid patients. The states that allow Medicaid direct payment pay NPs 80% to 100% of the amount paid to physicians billing for the same service. Currently, Congress is considering whether states should receive block grants whereby each state decides how to disburse their Medicaid funds. In this scenario, NPs may experience lower reimbursement rates than have been provided thus far.

Rural Health Clinics

Rural health clinics were established as a Medicare Part B and Medicaid service in 1977 to improve access to care in rural areas. This was the first time Medicare recognized the services of NPs without requiring the direct supervision of physicians. Prior to the passage of the Rural Health Clinic Services Act of 1977 (Public Law 95-210), midlevel practitioners (NPs, and PAs) were not eligible for reimbursement from Medicare or, in some states, from Medicaid. Congress recognized that midlevel practitioners were widely accepted in many communities, and payment for their services under public programs could result in greater incentives for them to practice in rural areas.

Amendments to the Act in 1987 increased the reimbursement cap for independent rural health clinics to $46, mandated future annual increases and linked them to the Medicare economic index. The amendment also added the services of clinical psychologists as reimbursable.

Amendments of 1989 to OBRA reduced the requirements related to the percentage of time midlevel practitioners were required to work in a certified rural health clinic from 60% to 50% of the time that the clinic is open. CNMs and clinical social work services were added to the group of midlevel practitioners who could be directly reimbursed for services in rural health clinics.

Amendments to the Rural Health Clinic Act in 1990 made further allowances to facilitate certification of rural health clinics, to waive employment requirements for midlevel practitioners if the clinics were experiencing recruiting difficulties, and other facilitating mechanisms to improve access to care for persons living in rural areas. In October 1990, there were 584 rural health clinics scattered throughout the United States, the number varying greatly among states.

A new Medicare physician fee schedule was enacted by Congress and became effective January 1, 1992. Under this schedule, Medicare continued to pay 80% of the allowed charge. The fee schedule amount for a service was calculated on the basis of three numbers: *relative value units*, which are established nationally for each procedure code and which do not vary among carriers; *geographic practice cost indices* (GPCI), based on the location of services rendered; and *national conversion factor*, which is a single national number used by all carriers in calculating payments under Medicare.

The physician fee schedule payments apply to physicians' services, services "incident to" physicians' services, outpatient physical therapy and occupational therapy services, diagnostic tests other than clinical laboratory tests, and radiology services. The fee schedule also applies regardless of whether the services are provided by a physician or nonphysician. In federally designated *health professional shortage areas* (HPSAs), physicians receive an additional 10% above the amount paid under the fee schedule. Anesthesia services are based on actual time as a factor in computing payments. The payment is determined by multiplying an *anesthesia conversion factor* adjusted by the locality GPCI by the sum of anesthesia base and time units.

Medicare payment for nonphysician practitioners is linked to the physician fee schedule for services rendered by NPs, CNMs, CNSs, CRNAs, and PAs. The rate of payment for CNMs is 65% of the physician fee; for NPs, the rate is 75% in hospital settings and 85% in nonhospital settings (NF, SNF); for PAs, the rate is 65% for both hospital and nonhospital settings and 75% for assistance in surgery. Unlike physicians, each nonphysician practitioner must accept Medicare assignment when they render any practitioner service. CRNAs were the first specialty nursing group to receive direct Medicare Part B reimbursement under OBRA 1986.

OBRA 1989 (Public Law 101–239) became effective April 1, 1990, and allowed the employer of an NP to submit claims to the Medicare carrier (in the state) for services rendered by the NP to a nursing home resident in a nursing facility (NF) or a skilled nursing facility (SNF). Eligible services were those which the NP was legally authorized to perform in accordance with state law or state nurse practice act. The NP had to work in collaboration with a physician. *Collaboration* was defined in *Medicare Carriers*

Manual instructions as "guidelines jointly developed by the NP and the physician that address medical direction and appropriate supervision."[3] The payment for NP services was limited to 85% of the participating-physician fee schedule amount for the comparable service. Claims for services were made on an assignment basis, that is, the NP's employer could not charge the nursing home resident beyond the Medicare-allowed fee. Only the employer (physician, hospital, NF, or SNF) of the NP could submit the claim for the service, and the claim had to be filed under the employer's Medicare Part B provider number obtained from a Medicare carrier. The employer could not be a group of incorporated NPs. The employer was required to withhold social security taxes from wages paid to an employee during the year and match the tax withheld from the employee's wages.

OBRA 1990 (Public Law 101–508), which became effective January 1, 1991, changed Medicare law to cover the services of NPs and CNSs in rural areas. The 1991 act allows NPs and CNSs to bill directly for services provided to nursing home residents in rural areas. The services of the NP and CNS must be delivered in collaboration with a physician. Eligible services are those Medicare-covered services that can be provided, according to state law or regulations, by an NP or a CNS. Claims for payment are submitted directly to the Medicare carrier by the NP or CNS, with the payment level of 75% of the participating-physician fee schedule for physician services performed in a hospital and 85% of the participating-physician fee schedule amount for all other services, including services delivered in nursing facilities. If the NP or CNS is employed by a nursing facility, hospital, or physician, they may sign over billing rights to the employer, with payment made on an assignment-related basis.

Federal Employees Health Benefits Program

The Federal Employees Health Benefits Program (FEHBP) is a voluntary contributory program open to all employees of the federal government. Through the various plans, employees are offered the opportunity to acquire for themselves and their families protection against the cost of health-care services, including services for prolonged illnesses or serious accidents. The benefits may be retained by employees after retirement. The federal government contributes to the cost of the plans, with employees paying their share through payroll deductions. Based on a 1982 law, federal employees and postal workers are covered by Medicare hospitalization insurance, for which they pay 1.45% of salary each biweekly period.

In the 99th Congress, legislation (Public Law 99–251) was enacted authorizing direct reimbursement for nonphysician providers, including registered nurses, in medically underserved areas. During the final days of the 101st Congress, Senator Daniel Inouye (D, Hawaii) attached an amendment to the Treasury, Postal Service Appropriations legislation that mandated direct reimbursement for APNs under FEHBP. The law (Public Law 101-509) was enacted to amend Section 8902(k)(1) of Title 5 of the United States Code, effective November 5, 1990, allowing federal employees enrolled in FEHBP health plans direct access to CNMs, NPs, and CNSs.

Civilian Health and Medical Program of the Uniformed Services

For 25 years, CHAMPUS has been a vital part of entitlements that members of the uniformed services have earned. This plan shares the cost of covered health care obtained by eligible members of military families from civilian sources when they cannot get care (or live too far) from a military hospital or clinic.

Worldwide, CHAMPUS processed about 18 million claims in 1992 and paid more than $3.5 billion in benefits for covered care. Claims for reimbursement may be filed by the patient, the patient's military sponsor, or the provider of care. The types of APNs who may provide covered care through CHAMPUS are CNPs and CPNs.

PRIVATE SOURCES OF REIMBURSEMENT

Fee-for-Service Payment

For a number of years, nurses have sought direct payment in terms of fee-for-service from private and public payers. Under the emerging changes in health-care reimbursements, particularly in managed care, the traditional fee-for-service payment system is virtually nonexistent. Payments from health insurance companies and plans will now be geared to the lowest cost per unit of care provided with the maximum of quality, according to the cost-benefit ratio.

The federal government's health-care insurance programs consider nurses, particularly APNs, as part of the federal plan for providing health care to all persons. Part of this consideration includes how nurses, NPs, NMWs, CNSs, CRNAs, and PAs will be reimbursed.

Private Companies

Many private health insurance plans are available to individuals and groups. APNs who are able to provide services under any insurance coverage plan, whether public or private, are required to obtain an identification number, such as a Drug Enforcement Agency (DEA) number from the federal government, to be eligible for direct reimbursement. (Psychiatric CNSs in private practice are not required to have a DEA number.) In addition, the APN must complete appropriate forms in a timely manner to receive payment. Once identified as a provider of care, APNs can bill individually directly to the private carrier for reimbursement for services.

Insurance policies that prevent APNs from being reimbursed directly reinforce the dominance of physicians, reduce collegial relationships, limit professional autonomy for nurses, limit consumer choice, and limit access to services, particularly for persons in underserved areas and among underserved, underinsured, or uninsured population groups. Many government officials and policy makers believe that fee-for-service reimbursement is inflationary because it encourages increased utilization and fee inflation. Officials also argue that APNs complement, rather than substitute for, physician services; thus, they should not be individually reimbursed. In addition, because, in theory, reimbursement enables APNs to be more independent, physicians and others argue against changes in established reimbursement patterns.

REFERENCES

1. Health Care Financing Administration. *Medicare Carriers Manual.* Claims Process: Transmittal 1421, May 1992; Claims Process: Transmittal 1422, April 1992. Baltimore: Health Care Financing Administration, 1992.
2. Human J, Van Hook RT. Preface to *Amendments to the Rural Health Services Act,* 1987.
3. Health Care Financing Administration. *Medicare Carriers Manual: Instructions on Claims Process.* Baltimore: Health Care Financing Administration, 1992.

BIBLIOGRAPHY

American Association of Nurse Anesthetists. *States Requiring Direct Private Insurance Reimbursement to CRNAs by Statute.* Park Ridge, IL: American Association of Nurse Anesthetists, 1991.
American Nurses' Association. *Medicaid Coverage.* Washington, DC: American Nurses' Association, Division of Governmental Affairs, 1992.
Bankert M. *Watchful Care: A History of America's Nurse Anesthetists.* New York: Continuum Publishing, 1989.
Health Care Financing Administration. *Understanding the Medicare Physician Fee Schedule and Related Practitioner Payments.* Baltimore: Health Care Financing Administration, November 1991.

————. *Medicaid: A Brief Summary of Title XIX of the Social Security Act.* Baltimore: Health Care Financing Administration, October 1991.

————. *Health Care Financing, Program Statistics: Medicare and Medicaid Data Book, 1990.* (HCFA Pub. No. 03314). Baltimore: Health Care Financing Administration, 1991.

Kongstvedt PR. *Essentials of Managed Health Care.* Gaithersburg, MD: Aspen Publishing, 1995.

Mittelstadt P. *The Reimbursement Manual.* Washington, DC: American Nurses Publishing, 1993.

Simonson DC, Garde JF. Reimbursement for clinical services. In Foster SC, Jordan LM, eds. *Professional Aspects of Nurse Anesthesia Practice.* Park Ridge, IL: American Association of Nurse Anesthetists, 1994: 129–142.

Stevens R. *In Sickness and in Wealth: American Hospitals in the Twentieth Century.* New York: Basic Books, 1989.

Federal Laws

Deficit Reduction Act of 1984 (PL 98-369).

Office of Rural Health Policy. *The Rural Health Clinic Services Act* (PL 95-210). Rockville, MD: National Rural Health Association, Office of Rural Health Policy, Health Resources and Services Administration, Public Health Service, U.S. Department of Health and Human Services, January 1991.

Omnibus Budget Reconciliation Act of 1986 (PL 99-509), Washington, DC: U.S. Government Printing Office, 1988.

Omnibus Budget Reconciliation Act of 1987 (PL 100-203), Washington, DC: U.S. Government Printing Office, 1989.

Omnibus Budget Reconciliation Act of 1989 (PL 101-239), *Federal Register,* June 29, 1991. Washington, DC: U.S. Government Printing Office.

Omnibus Budget Reconciliation Act of 1990 (PL 101-508), effective January 1, 1991. Washington, DC: U.S. Government Printing Office.

Social Security Amendments of 1983 (PL 98-21).

Tax Equity and Fiscal Responsibility Act of 1982 (PL 97-248).

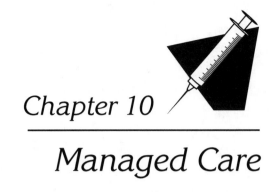

Chapter 10

Managed Care

Description
Philosophy and Goals
Effects on Advanced Practice Nurses

Health care in the United States is undergoing substantial change. Health care has become "Big Business"—capable of consuming and controlling every aspect of health-care access, quality, delivery, and professional and support staffs. Many people and employees see this type of ownership and administration as a way of stabilizing and maintaining hospitals, particularly the smaller community hospitals, of providing jobs, and guaranteeing more equal care. At the present time, managed care, which many have dubbed "managed costs," is almost universally in place. Physicians work in group practices, often under the direction and management of the hospital in which the individual physicians, who had worked in solo practices, had privileges for many years. The hospitals or the large, private health maintenance organizations (HMOs) manage the budget and accounting and billing procedures. Rapidly expanding private hospital ownership groups (such as Columbia Health, which began in Texas with the purchase of two hospitals and has grown to an $18 billion business and the ownership of hundreds more hospitals, with an additional hospital being bought nearly every 10 days) have become mammoth HMOs that could likely become monopolies, controlling completely all the health-care delivery in the United States—perhaps in the world. Wherever managed care occurs, the concern is cost of care; therefore, managed care is seen as Big Business because of the profit motive behind the system.

DESCRIPTION

Descriptions of managed care vary. There is no single, uniformly accepted descriptor that defines a managed care organizational structure. The term has been applied to a wide range of prepayment arrangements, negotiated discounts, and agreements for prior authorizations and audits of performance of all health-care providers. The fee-for-service model that had been in place for decades is replaced by a system in which all service items have a designated maximum charge, regardless of who provides the services. This method of payment by insurance companies is adopted in order to project costs of services, and to standardize costs for services in all health-care settings. Thus, in most HMOs, direct reimbursement to providers has become a thing of the past; most providers are salaried by the HMO.

Although all physicians are moving into group practices, not all are salaried employees of large hospitals or giant corporations. Some physicians have created their own groups, preferred provider organizations (PPOs), which operate as miniature versions of HMOs—the members of the group share revenues, and visits are costed out. Other PPOs operate under the fiscal management of a hospital or another health-care entity.

A common thread running through all the variations is that some type of restriction is imposed under some type of binding contractual arrangement on fee-for-service. In addition, within the group practices and HMOs, costs are maintained within very rigid parameters, and care is rationed to a greater extent than it has been in the past. For example, elective surgery patients are being moved farther down on the wait list, and limits are being placed on the extent of use of costly diagnostic testing and treatment.

Insurance companies decide which services, medications, specialists, and hospitalizations are covered under their health-care plans. Allowable services are perceived in terms of cost savings over the paid period of insurance; quality of services is not a consideration. Cost-effective care is the focus, and cost overshadows all decisions made by providers. From a different perspective, therefore, managed care is considered a method of rationing care at a fixed price.

PHILOSOPHY AND GOALS

HMOs advocate health promotion and disease prevention. Healthy people do not need care, and problems are seen and diagnosed at an early stage, which precludes lengthy and costly treatment of disease at advanced stages. Managed care systems benefit by keeping patients well, and providing care at the earliest phase of an illness episode. Patients prefer this kind of care, because it usually results in fewer lost days of work, less severe illness, and a feeling that they are being cared for at every stage, not just when they are sickest.

A goal of managed care is to modify the behavior of both consumers and providers through financial penalties and rewards. The process has been termed "micro-costing." Providers who order the fewest laboratory tests and consistently require the lowest payment for services, while delivering quality care, are rewarded by means of a bonus system from the HMO with which they are associated. The goal is not simply to lower costs, but to ensure that maximum value is received from the resources used in the production and delivery of health-care services to the population. Managed care therefore affects all care providers, results in more equitable financial rewards for providers, and provides better services for consumers, all at the lowest possible cost.

Currently, about one in five U.S. citizens belongs to an HMO, at a specified monthly or annual cost, which allows the patient to choose a provider from a list of selected providers. The HMO pays the provider either a monthly salary to see a specific number of patients each day, or a monthly capitated (per capita) fee per patient, with payment made to the provider on a monthly basis. The payment fee per patient varies.

However, the number of patients seen per provider is a critical factor in maintaining employment. "Productivity measures," such as total number of patient-visits per year, play an increasing role in how HMOs and other types of care facilities evaluate health-care providers. Providers who can show the larger number of patient visits per year fare well; those who do not measure up to certain levels may be let go. Finances therefore rule the health-care roost for the foreseeable future and will likely remain the strongest of forces forever.

EFFECTS ON ADVANCED PRACTICE NURSES

Mainly because of the changing method of payment, employment of nurses is undergoing the most significant changes since the 1950s. Only a small percentage of advanced practice nurses (APNs) have engaged in private practice; in the largest states, the proportion of APNs in solo practice is 5% or less. Under managed care, the percentage is likely to decrease.

Many APNs employed by HMOs find the situation satisfactory because of the regular guaranteed salary and the often substantial benefits. In addition, APNs function at a very high level when providing wellness counseling and health promotion, and patients' satisfaction with

APN care is always excellent in this regard. HMOs also support continuing education for their health-care providers, more than that supported in most private practice settings because practices that have smaller numbers of staff cannot afford to have practitioners away for education programs lest the practice be short-staffed, perhaps causing patients to be turned away.

There are disadvantages, however, especially for APNs who are accustomed to spend time with patients to provide education and information. The demanding schedule that most HMOs expect providers to meet requires that patient visits be limited to 15 minutes, sometimes 10 minutes. This schedule limits the quality of care and patient services that can be offered, and certainly limits the role of the APN. Providers can be sanctioned for making too many referrals, prescribing a medication or treatment not on the approved list (overutilization), for taking longer than the allotted time with each patient, and for extending the length of patients' hospitalizations.

Not all HMOs want APNs on their staff. Much depends on the organization's history and whether there has been a mix of providers in the past. However, with cost savings in the forefront, even somewhat reluctant HMOs may begin to look with favor on APNs who are not only experts in their fields, but who are also cost-effective.

Physicians who have worked with APNs are favorably disposed toward them, but the large, professional medical organizations, both state and national, are opposed. APNs are seen by these organizations as a threat to physicians in the face of shrinking financial rewards. To continue to be a part of emerging managed care, APNs must make certain that they are listed with a specified managed care organization as a designated primary care provider (PCP), rather than working with physicians in a clinic situation in which only the physician is listed as a PCP, even though the APN does actual caregiving.

At this point, it is difficult to predict the changes that will occur as a result of reengineering within every health-care setting. All APNs need to know how the system is changing, what economic trends are occurring, and where APNs fit into the picture. APNs will likely reap some benefits and lose out in some areas under managed care; this is true for all providers. However, the advent of managed care means that APNs also have to become more involved in the political processes, both locally and nationally. For example, APNs in some states have tried to have legislators incorporate the terms *any willing provider* or *health-care provider* as the preferred terms, rather than *physician,* in nurse practice acts describing scope of practice because the turf battles will continue and perhaps escalate as reimbursement payments become leaner and patients continue to be dropped from Medicaid and, perhaps, Medicare systems.

Because of their cost-effective, quality care, most HMOs and other managed care organizations are likely to want APNs on their staffs. Experts do not predict any change in employment opportunities in these settings.

BIBLIOGRAPHY

Barer ML, Evans RG, Holt M, Morrison JL. It ain't necessarily so: The cost implications of health care reform. *Health Aff*, Fall:88–99, 1994.

Hastings K. Health care reform: We need it but do we have the national will to shape our future? *Nurse Practitioner*, 20(1):52, 1994.

Hicks LL, Stallmeyer JM, Coleman JR. *Role of the Nurse in Managed Care*. Washington DC: American Nurses Publishing, 1993.

Kongstvedt PR. *Essentials of Managed Health Care*. Gaithersburg, MD: Aspen Publishing, 1995.

Managed care: NPs work to weather the changes. *NPNews*, 3(1):5, 1995.

Pearson LA. Annual update of how each state stands on legislative issues affecting advanced nurse practice. *Nurse Practitioner*, 21(1):10–70, 1996.

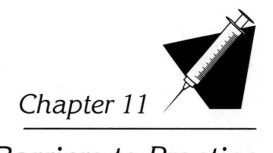

Chapter 11

Barriers to Practice

Today, more than ever perhaps, advanced practice nurses (APNs) are besieged on every side by other health-care professional groups, various professional organizations, and federal and state legislative actions regarding managed care. Forces that address containment of costs, quality of care, leadership status ("captain of the ship"), downsizing or reengineering within health-care facilities, and the economic crisis in the United States impinge on the practice of APNs, particularly APN groups—nurse practitioners (NPs), certified nurse-midwives (CNMs), and certified registered nurse anesthetists (CRNAs)—whose work requires responsibility for performing services in areas of practice that traditionally have been considered the domain of physicians.

ADVANCED PRACTICE NURSES

Physician and nursing groups have argued for many years about the term "supervision." The majority of APNs prefer to work collaboratively with physicians, rather than totally independently and without consultation and collaboration with physicians.

In June 1995, the American Medical Association (AMA) House of Delegates, after hearing debate about advanced nursing practice, voted to adopt a resolution calling for tighter restrictions on NP practice, including physician supervision in all practice settings, a stand that fails to recognize that APNs are independently licensed professionals responsible and accountable for their own practice. The AMA's resolution appears to take a definitive stance. The guidelines adopted by the AMA state:[1]

1. The physician is responsible for the supervision of nurse practitioners and other advanced practice nurses in all settings.
2. The physician is responsible for managing the health care of patients in all practice settings.
3. Health-care services delivered in an integrated practice must be within the scope of each practitioner's professional license, as defined by state law.
4. In an integrated practice with a nurse practitioner, the physician is responsible for supervising and coordinating care and, with the appropriate input of the nurse practitioner, ensuring the quality of health care provided to patients.
5. The extent of involvement by the nurse practitioner in initial assessment, and implementation of treatment will depend on the complexity and acuity of the patient's condition, as determined by the supervising/collaborating physician.
6. The role of the nurse practitioner in the delivery of care in an integrated practice should be defined through mutually agreed upon written practice protocols, job descriptions, and written contracts.
7. These practice protocols should delineate the appropriate involvement of the two professionals in the care of patients, based on the complexity and acuity of the patient's condition.
8. At least one physician in the integrated practice must be immediately available at all times for supervision and consultation when needed by the nurse practitioner.
9. Patients are to be made clearly aware at all times whether they are being cared for by a physician or a nurse practitioner.
10. In an integrated practice, there should be a professional and courteous relationship between physician and nurse practitioner, with mutual acknowledgement of, and respect for, each other's contributions to patient care.
11. Physicians and nurse practitioners should review and document, on a regular basis, the care of all patients with whom the nurse practitioner is involved. Physicians and nurse practitioners must work closely enough together to become fully conversant with each other's practice patterns.

Also at this meeting, in separate action, the AMA House of Delegates adopted Resolution 320, which calls for the AMA to study the use of nonphysician health-care providers in medical practice with regard to

(1) quality assurance and overall impact on quality of care, (2) practice oversight and regulation, (3) the effect on health-care costs, and (4) financial implications for physician practices, both individually and collectively.[2] In hospitals, APNs must, like physicians, be granted practice privileges to be a member of the interdisciplinary team in a particular hospital. The requirements for privileges are generally developed by the hospital's medical staff through bylaws. However, in some cases, restrictive bylaws prevent APNs from practicing to the full extent of their professional capability and authority, as granted by state licensing laws. For example, some hospitals have exclusive contracts with specialty physician groups, such as anesthesiologists, thus effectively shutting out CRNAs.

NURSE-MIDWIVES

Concern about "territorial rights" has also produced competition between CNMs and physicians. Colman McCarthy, a journalist with *The Washington Post* and an outspoken advocate of nurse-midwifery, wrote an editorial (January 16, 1996) about a meeting of the obstetricians associated with the hospitals of the New York Health and Hospitals Association. The obstetricians were addressing the quality of care provided by the hundreds of CNMs who practice within this group of hospitals. McCarthy states [partially paraphrased]:[3]

> When physicians begin to be nervous about their turf being threatened, they introduce "quality of care" and "patient safety." When shown reams of data from many studies about the high-level care of nurse-midwives, the response is, "Show me more data"; there is never enough data to show that nurse-midwives provide outstanding care to thousands of women and babies every year. Granted, nurse-midwives deliver essentially healthy women, although many deliver adolescents who are considered a high-risk group, and drug-addicted and AIDS patients, also considered high-risk. Their patients practically never sue them, because they are satisfied with the care they and their babies receive. Of deliveries performed in the New York City hospitals last year, almost 30% were delivered by nurse-midwives. However, in Europe and Australia, 75% of women are delivered by midwives as a matter of tradition and acceptance. Now, under managed care, payments to physicians, obstetricians, and other care providers, are lower. The cost of malpractice liability insurance for obstetricians is expensive ($35,000 or more per year). Thus, many obstetricians want to deliver healthy, low-risk women, not just those who are high-risk or who have complications such as diabetes and

hypertension. Both numbers and economics play roles in the situation. As more women elect to have nurse-midwives deliver their babies, fewer seek care from obstetricians.

In a response to McCarthy's editorial, Ralph W. Hale, Executive Director of the American College of Obstetricians and Gynecologists, provided a cogent, realistic perspective: "There's no argument that nurse-midwives are an important and vital part of obstetrical care." He points out that gender is not an issue, since "the majority of young OB/GYNs today are women." He admonishes, "Let's work together to improve our health care system—not perpetuate myths. . . ."[4] The University of Maryland Hospital, Baltimore, for example, has both an obstetrical service and a nurse-midwifery service, thereby allowing patients to choose a preferred provider. This collaborative relationship demonstrates that care by OB/GYNs and NMWs should be complementary, not competitive.

NURSE ANESTHETISTS

Barriers also exist for CRNAs in their practice. In 1982, the Tax Equity and Fiscal Responsibility Act (TEFRA) established the criteria that an anesthesiologist must meet to be paid by Medicare for medically directing CRNAs. The anesthesiologist was expected to:

- perform a preanesthesia examination and evaluation
- prescribe the anesthesia plan
- personally participate in the most demanding procedures of the anesthesia plan, including induction and emergence
- ensure that any procedure in the anesthesia plan that the anesthesiologist did not perform, was performed by a qualified anesthetist
- monitor the course of anesthesia administration at intervals
- remain physically present and available for immediate diagnosis and treatment of emergency events
- provide indicated postanesthesia care

The TEFRA payment conditions came about because of abuses to the system by some anesthesiologists who were making huge profits by billing for supervising CRNAs when the anesthesiologists were not present or in the hospital. The purpose of the payment conditions, therefore, was to place anesthesiologists in positions of accountability for the services they were claiming to provide as they worked with or employed CRNAs.

Unfortunately, the TEFRA conditions have been inappropriately interpreted as quality-of-care standards, rather than conditions for reimbursement of physicians. As a result, the TEFRA conditions have led to restrictions of CRNA practice by not allowing CRNAs to perform all the components of an anesthesia service that they are legally authorized to carry out. Some anesthesiologists insist on performing all anesthesia inductions themselves, thus disallowing the CRNA from performing all aspects of anesthesia care. In addition, disruption in the flow of cases through surgical schedules has occurred because the entire surgical team must wait for the availability of an anesthesiologist to start or end a case, even though the CRNA is capable of doing the procedures.

The TEFRA conditions also have put into place a system that requires and pays for duplicative services, such as requiring the anesthesiologist to do a preanesthesia examination and evaluation, which the CRNA must do again for personal knowledge about the case and the need for documentation. Duplications in aspects of care are costly, in both time and money.

In several states, physician-controlled insurance companies have attempted to restrict the practice of CRNAs by adopting restrictive endorsements that require surgeons to follow certain procedures when working with CRNAs; the restrictions are based on statements that imply additional liability when a surgeon works with a CRNA. Ignorance of the quality of care given by CRNAs may contribute to misjudgments. However, outcome data comparing care by anesthesiologists and that by CRNAs do not support allegations that CRNAs give lower-quality care. Some physician-controlled insurance companies also charge higher premiums because their physicians employ or supervise CRNAs; their rationale for higher premiums is perplexing, since other insurance companies not controlled by physicians neither charge higher premiums nor include restrictive endorsements on physicians who work with CRNAs.

The American Society of Anesthesiologists (ASA) issued guidelines for obstetric anesthesia that state: "Regional anesthesia should be initiated by a physician with appropriate privileges and maintained by or under the medical direction of such an individual."[5] This statement, issued about *obstetric* anesthesia, clearly is intended to restrict the practice of CRNAs regarding the administration of regional anesthesia in maternity cases, although the stated intent was to provide safer anesthesia care for all patients. Patient outcome data have consistently shown that the anesthesia care provided by CRNAs is of the same high quality as that given by anesthesiologists.

CLINICAL NURSE SPECIALISTS

CNSs experience the same barriers to practice that all APNs face, depending on their area of specialization, degree of autonomy, and relationships with other health-care professionals, employers, and patients. Barriers come in the form of restricted practice, inability to obtain prescriptive authority because of state legislation, and isolation from other health professionals who can provide support.

SUMMARY

Advanced practice nurses need to work together to inform consumers, state and national legislators, health insurance companies, other health professionals, and employers about the scope of their practice under the law and document their qualifications to practice at a specific level by credentials, certification, and standards of practice. Education and a spirit of cooperation and inclusion can pave the way to smooth interprofessional relationships and provide opportunities for APNs to practice their specialties at the appropriate level.

REFERENCES

1. American Medical Association Board of Trustees. *Model Guidelines for Physician and Nurse Practitioner Integrated Practice* (Report 6-A-95). Chicago: American Medical Association, 1995.
2. AMA adopts resolutions that attempt to restrict NP practice. *NPNews*, 3(5):2, 1995.
3. McCarthy C. The case for nurse-midwives. *The Washington Post*, January 16, 1996: C-6.
4. Hale RE. Response to "The case for nurse-midwives." *The Washington Post*, January 20, 1996: A-22.
5. American Society of Anesthesiologists. *ASA Guidelines for Regional Anesthesia for Obstetrics* and *ASA Statement on the Anesthesia Care Team*. Park Ridge, IL: American Society of Anesthesiologists, 1992.

BIBLIOGRAPHY

American Association of Nurse Anesthetists. *Barriers to Nurse Anesthesia Practice.* Park Ridge, IL: American Association of Nurse Anesthetists, 1993.
Blumenreich GA, Wolf BL. Restrictions on CRNAs imposed by physician-controlled insurance companies. *Am Assoc Nurse Anesthesiol J* 54:538–539, 1986.
Medicare Regulations 405–552. *Conditions for Payment: Anesthesiology Services*, Vol. 4. Chicago: Commerce Clearinghouse, 1992: 7930.

Chapter 12

Malpractice

National Practitioner Data Bank
Litigation
Summary

NATIONAL PRACTITIONER DATA BANK

The National Practitioner Data Bank (NPDB) was established by the federal government in 1990 as a depository for health-care providers' malpractice payments by insurers and adverse actions by licensing boards, hospitals, or professional societies. The purpose of the NPDB is to prevent possibly incompetent practitioners against whom malpractice claims have been made from moving from the state in which the malpractice claim was made to another state and continuing to practice. The NPDB therefore monitors providers' activities with regard to liability claims and payments. Malpractice payments are required to be reported to the NPDB regardless of the settlement amount. A report by the insurer is made when the payment is based on a written claim of clinical malpractice and names individual providers and organizations that are involved in the liability suit.

The NPDB must be checked by any hospital initially granting clinical privileges and every two years thereafter. Access to the NPDB is limited to specified individuals and agencies: a plaintiff's attorney on a per case basis, hospitals, state licensing boards, other health-care entities, professional societies, and providers may request access to their own files.

The NPDB data show that nurses have less than 3% of the reported malpractice payments; while physicians have over 97% in two 17.5-month periods. Data about nurses are grouped according to information in Tables 12–1 and 12–2.[1] These data show that the payment report rate for physicians is more than twice that for all categories of nurses and advanced

TABLE 12–1
Malpractice payments

Type of Practitioner	No. of Practitioners	*Sept. 1990–Feb. 1992*		
		No. of Reports	No. of Reports per 1000 Practitioners
Physician	544,490	17,775	32.6
RN	1,582,816	334	0.2
CRNA	16,831	112	6.7
NMW	2886	16	5.5
NP	20,649	20	1.0
All nurses	1,627,000	482	0.3

Source: Birkholz G. Malpractice data from the National Practitioner Data Bank. *Nurse Practitioner* 20:32–35, 1995.

TABLE 12–2
Malpractice payments

Type of Practitioner	No. of Practitioners	*Mar. 1992–July 1993*		
		No. of Reports	No. of Reports per 1000 Practitioners
Physician	560,775	21,350	38
RN	1,807,703	354	0.2
CRNA	18,617	126	6.8
NMW	3045	23	7.6
NP	23,659	14	0.6
All nurses	1,853,024	517	0.3

Source: Birkholz G. Malpractice data from the National Practitioner Data Bank. *Nurse Practitioner* 20:32–35, 1995.

practice nurses (APNs) combined. If malpractice claim payment is used as a satisfaction indicator, these data support the statement that patients are more satisfied with APN care than with physician care. Report rates for CRNAs and CNMs are higher, primarily because these practitioners provide care that is more invasive and more technologically sophisticated than that used by nurse practitioners (NPs). Certified nurse specialists are generally employees of health-care facilities and are therefore not implicated as individuals or specific providers in malpractice suits, which are most often brought against hospitals, physicians, and nurses. Important to note, however, is that malpractice payment reports are not malpractice settlement claims. There is no requirement that any breach-of-care standard be *proven* for reporting to the NPDB; allegations and findings of malpractice are reported. However, the reports do represent patient dissatisfaction with the providers care, and willingness of the insurer to pay in response to the patient's claim.

Providers and others using the NPDB need to know that there is underreporting and that claims are about 5 to 8 years old. The physician rate is underrepresented because of elimination of physicians during claim negotiations, and the lack of duty by named government and private health-care entities to identify unnamed providers. One implication for APNs is that they need to be aware of peer review processes that attempt to identify individuals who should be reported to the NPDB, particularly if the peer review group is composed primarily of physicians.

LITIGATION

Beckmann[2] lists the most common adverse malpractice outcomes regarding *registered nurses,* not nurse practitioners. However, several of the causes (listed below) of adverse outcomes could apply to APNs as well, such as:

- inadequate [or incomplete] nursing assessment
- medication administration error
- inadequate [or delayed] communication with the physician regarding patient status
- inadequate care by the physician

What occurs often is that, in the case of a hospitalized patient who alleges injury from inadequate care given during his or her hospital stay, the patient files a lawsuit, citing the hospital and all physicians, nurses, and "others" who were involved in direct care. The hospital and all persons named would be included as defendants; the patient is the plaintiff. In these cases, no individual health professional is identified as the one causing the injury; all share equal responsibility. The hospital pays the costs if the court rules in favor of the plaintiff.

The following are two examples of malpractice cases brought against individual APNs:

Case 1.   An obstetrics/gynecology nurse practitioner sees a patient who comes to the clinic for the first time and states that she thinks she is pregnant, but who had a spontaneous abortion occur the previous day. The NP obtains a complete history and performs a physical including a pelvic examination. She tells the patient that she likely expressed the products of conception and that the vaginal bleeding should stop within a week. The NP orders routine laboratory blood and urine tests, including a quantitative serum human chorionic gonadotropin (hCG) pregnancy test. She reassures the patient that the pregnancy has been expelled and that she should be fine.

Ten days later, the patient returns and says the bleeding has not stopped and she is experiencing some lower abdominal cramping. The NP examines her and tells her the bleeding will likely stop in a few more days.

Four days later, the patient returns. She now has a fever of 102°F, and the NP observes that the vaginal discharge has a foul odor. The NP asks the clinic physician to evaluate the patient. The physician finds that the patient is febrile, with an acute pelvic infection and possible retained products of conception in the uterus. He orders a quantitative serum hCG on an emergency basis and a urinalysis. The hCG report indicates that the patient is still pregnant. The patient is immediately hospitalized and undergoes a procedure to evacuate the uterus completely. She receives intravenous antibiotics to resolve the infection. She is hospitalized for 7 days, after which the IV antibiotics are discontinued, but oral antibiotics are prescribed for another week after discharge.

The patient sued the NP for malpractice and damages; the court ruled in favor of the plaintiff.

The NP did not provide adequate follow-up care for the patient. One major fault being that the NP should have ordered sequential hCGs, which would have gradually decreased if the pregnancy had been completely aborted. Having failed to do this, she was found guilty of malpractice and her license was suspended for 1 year.

Case 2. A nurse practitioner is on duty in the hospital one evening, as a member of the house staff. A patient is brought to the unit from the emergency room. Two hours earlier he sustained a fractured tibia in a motorcycle accident and had been given emergency treatment and a cast was applied in the ER. Several hours later, the patient begins complaining of pain in the injured leg. The prescribed medication is not sufficiently potent to relieve the pain. The NP notices that there is some swelling in the patient's toes. She places an immediate call to the orthopedist on duty, who is now at another hospital in response to an emergency call. The NP calls the second orthopedist on call; his answering machine indicates that he is unavailable. The NP leaves her name and the telephone number of the unit. She asks the unit clerk if either orthopedist has beeper numbers; the clerk says that she had not been given access to them. The NP then calls the house officer for the hospital, but he is in the operating room. She checks the patient again, gives him a second dose of pain medication, notes that his toes look a little dusky in color, and that the edema has increased slightly. She asks the unit clerk to locate a cast cutter and calls the orthopedists and the house officer again.

The orthopedist on first call arrives at the hospital 2 hours later and has the patient moved to the operating room and put under quarantine conditions. When he removes the cast, he recognizes that the patient has developed gas gangrene, which is caused by anaerobic bacteria, later identified as *Clostridium perfringens*. Treatment requires open reduction of the tibial fracture and intravenous antibiotics for 14 days. The surgical wound has to remain open and some postoperative debridement is necessary on the first day. The patient has to be hospitalized for 2 weeks in a private room, under strict isolation conditions.

The patient subsequently sued the NP, claiming that she had not acted quickly enough in calling for assistance, resulting in greater pain, surgery, and a longer hospital stay.

The NP in this case acted as quickly as she could, called at least three physicians, all of whom were unavailable initially. She repeated the calls at short intervals, leaving a message each time. Fortunately, a highly qualified orthopedist arrived on the scene first and could proceed quickly with surgery and the appropriate follow-up treatment. The court ruled that she had acted as promptly as possible, although the hospital and the orthopedist were required to pay the plaintiff a total of $50,000.

Beckmann[2] reported that the number of malpractice cases against nurses working in hospitals increased almost 100% between 1976 and 1987. As more NPs take positions as house (physician) staff, the number of malpractice lawsuits against them are likely to increase. This increase in the number of malpractice cases corresponds to the increase in the level of acuity (of illness) among hospitalized patients, and the development of medical technology. Today, with most major academic teaching hospitals initiating reengineering strategies to cut costs, including using unlicensed technical assistants (UTAs) in place of nurses and reducing the number of specialist physicians to manage patients who are extremely sick, incidents of various kinds that may instigate malpractice claims are likely to increase. The cause is not the inadequacies of staff but the lack qualified health professionals to manage the increasing number of very ill patients in hospitals and in home care. Nurses who are well-educated and experienced are being let go and are being replaced by UTAs or, worse still, by hospital staff from housekeeping or maintenance departments who are given short first-aid and nursing care courses of 1 to 3 months, to take over the responsibilities once held exclusively by RNs.[3]

Recently, as part of reengineering strategies, some adjustments in the delivery of care and home care have improved the safe care of patients to some degree. Other reengineering strategies include the division of responsibilities for nurses and support personnel, and increased crosstraining to provide nurses with the skills needed to enable them to manage patients who are severely ill.

Advanced practice nurses are also becoming more attuned to the rapidly changing health-care system and are taking steps to strengthen and support their own knowledge and skill base in order to avoid malpractice suits.

SUMMARY

All APNs must be aware of the legal implications of practicing at a more autonomous level, to be responsible for all aspects of care, and to be accountable for their own clinical decisions and actions, both oral and written. A major aspect of "defensive" care is documentation of the care provided; detailed patient assessment information; times at which communications with staff members are initiated and responded to; precise information about medications ordered and given; and frequent, comprehensive reports regarding patients' status. An essential aspect of advanced practice is to know and to act within accepted standards of practice; lawsuits are generally brought against APNs who perform procedures or actions that are clearly, under a state's nurse practice act, outside the domain of advanced practice. Individual APNs need to keep a record of all credentials earned, continuing education programs attended, and experience with patients.

Today, because many APNs and physicians are entering into contractual agreements around group practice, the APN needs to read all contracts carefully; ask for clarification on issues that may be obscure; determine the honesty and integrity of all care providers in the group; and recognize the frequency and costs in time, effort, and money of malpractice suits. In providing care, APNs must be aware that using terms that are inconsistent with their field of expertise may be fuel for the person intent on making a malpractice claim; words, such as "counseling" or "cognitive/physical therapy," may lead others to assume that the APN is claiming to have credentials and skills that, in fact, she or he does not have. Most important of all is for the APN to be thoroughly familiar with both the state's nurse practice act and the medical practice act, to be better able to determine the difference in the scope of practice of each.

Most care providers are uncomfortable with the concept of defensive practice, as this relates to avoiding malpractice lawsuits. But today's health-care environment, and the fact that many people are looking for any words or actions on which to base a malpractice claim, make it necessary for all APNs to use all means available to protect themselves from being the target of a patient's malpractice suit.

REFERENCES

1. Birkholz G. Malpractice data from the National Practitioner Data Bank. *Nurse Practitioner,* 20(3):32–35, 1995.
2. Beckmann JP. *Nursing Negligence: Analyzing Malpractice in the Hospital Setting.* Thousand Oaks, CA: Sage, 1996.
3. Gordon S. What nurses stand for. *The Atlantic Monthly,* 279(2):80–82, 84–88, 1997.

Part IV

Current Issues and Trends

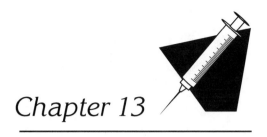

Chapter 13

Merging Nurse Practitioner and Clinical Nurse Specialist Roles

Since 1992, a developing trend among some nurse educators has been to merge the roles of clinical nurse specialist (CNS) and nurse practitioner (NP). The common misperception, even among nurse educators and practicing nurses, is that the roles are almost the same and that CNSs need take only an advanced physical assessment course and perhaps a pharmacology course to update their knowledge about drugs to qualify for the NP certifying examination.

This is a simplistic view of what NPs must know and apply, but there are many similarities in the two roles. The strengths that both groups have can be merged to produce a well-rounded advanced practice nurse (APN). The roles were notably different in the past, because CNSs practiced primarily in hospitals and NPs practiced in primary care settings. Today, CNSs practice in all settings, and NPs are increasingly found in acute care settings—hospitals and home health care. The trend towards CNSs and NPs practicing in the broad health-care arena, rather than specifically in one setting, is likely to continue into the next decade.

The educational preparation of CNSs and NPs is the same in basic knowledge and core courses such as nursing theory, research and statistics, pathophysiology, health promotion and disease prevention, and needs of the underserved population. APN education would be improved if a practical and efficient curriculum were developed to include all basic knowledge, skills, and core courses, with only the specialty areas requiring separate courses and clinical experience. From the merging of curriculums, new concepts and roles could develop, marking a new era for nursing education, research, and practice.

In December 1994, the American Association of Colleges of Nursing sponsored a Master's Education Conference in San Antonio, Texas, to facilitate open discussion, primarily among CNS and NP faculty, regarding the feasibility of merging the educational programs of the two specialties. The goal of the conference was to arrive at a consensus regarding direction for the programs. A majority was in favor of merging the programs, although the two sides of the issue were evident.

ARGUMENTS FOR MERGING

The following statements, taken from conference proceedings and studies of the roles of the two specialties, represent the main views favoring merger:

> [T]he practice patterns, legal and professional regulation, and education of nurses at the graduate level should be so aligned that one educational product, the advanced practice nurse, can fill a variety of roles in the health care system (Linda R. Cronenwett, PhD, Director of Research and Education, Dartmouth-Hitchcock Medical Center, Lebanon, NH).[1]

> A conscious decision by the profession to fold together clinician and practitioner preparation and practice roles would give nursing the initiative and control that will be lost if developments occur because of inattention or of vested interests. The merger of advanced practice roles would simplify the concept for consumers and practice sites; take advantage of the demand in acute care settings; and enable practitioners to follow patients through various settings.[2]

> Many similarities already exist in roles.

> Practice settings for both are expanding and overlapping.

> Unity and an increase in numbers would give more power to advanced practice nurses.

> Many similarities already exist in educational preparation.

> Increased cost effectiveness for colleges and universities would result if the roles were combined.

> Graduates with both credentials would be more marketable.[3]

ARGUMENTS AGAINST MERGING

Faculty against merging the two roles object primarily because of the possibility that the term *nurse practitioner* will disappear, replaced by APN. NPs have worked for many years to be recognized for their expertise. Members of Congress and their staffs, and many other significant groups, now know the term, what it means, and that NPs have provided quality, cost-effective care to people of all ages for over 30 years. If NPs were no longer known by the title, their identity would be lost.

> Scope of practice remains different, as typically NPs are generalists in promoting health and CNSs are acute care subspecialists.
>
> Legal entanglements exist with trying to include CNSs in existing advanced practice legislation.
>
> Titling (e.g., name recognition) and legal issues. NPs are widely recognized, particularly by members of Congress and state legislatures.
>
> Graduate programs would need to be longer, adversely affecting enrollment.[1]

Both internal and external forces are influencing the future direction of APN education: costs, number of qualified faculty, health-care needs, rapidly evolving areas such as scientific knowledge and technology, and the health-care delivery environment.[4]

SUMMARY

The question of whether to merge the CNS and NP roles at the master's degree educational level, is still being debated. Many issues—political, legislative, and educational—remain to be discussed and resolved. The major goal of all nursing education is to provide quality care to patients at the lowest cost.

Nothing is happening. In the APN programs at Johns Hopkins, for example, developed to prepare graduates as both CNSs and NPs, the CNS portion has been abandoned: the programs now prepare adult, pediatric, acute/critical care, and OB/GYN *nurse practitioners.*

REFERENCES

1. American Association of Colleges of Nursing. *Role of Differentiation of the Nurse Practitioner and Clinical Nurse Specialist: Reaching Toward Consensus.* Proceedings of the Master's Education Conference, San Antonio, TX, December 8–10, 1994. Washington, DC: American Association of Colleges of Nursing, 1995.
2. Hahn MS. Identity crisis? *Advances for Nurse Practitioners* 3(6):22–26, 49, 1995.
3. Mezey MD, McGivern DO. *Nurses, Nurse Practitioners: Evolution to Advanced Practice.* New York: Springer, 1993.
4. Soehren PM, Schumann LL. Enhanced role opportunities available to the CNS/nurse practitioner. *Clin Nurs Spec* 8:123–27, 1994.

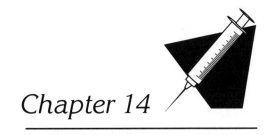

Chapter 14

State Legislative Issues

Title Protection and Scope of Practice
Prescriptive Authority

Each state has its own stand on legislation affecting nursing practice. Two categories of particular interest to advanced practice nurses (APNs) are title protection/scope of practice and prescriptive authority. (A third category, reimbursement, is discussed in Chapter 10.)

TITLE PROTECTION AND SCOPE OF PRACTICE

Twenty-five states and the District of Columbia have APN title protection, and the state Board of Nursing is the sole authority for scope of practice; there are no requirements for physician collaboration or supervision. The states are listed below. Asterisk (*) indicates that certified nurse specialists (CNSs) are not included.

Alaska	Kansas	Oregon*
Arkansas	Maine	Rhode Island*
Colorado	Michigan	Texas
Connecticut	Montana	Utah
Delaware	New Hampshire	Vermont
District of Columbia	New Mexico	Washington
Hawaii	North Dakota	West Virginia
Indiana	Oklahoma	Wyoming
Iowa		

Fifteen states have APN title protection, and the state Board of Nursing is the sole authority on scope of practice; in these states, physician collaboration or supervision is required. The states are listed below. Asterisk (*) indicates that CNSs are not included; double asterisks (**) indicate that only psychiatric/mental health CNSs are included.

Alabama	Kentucky	Nevada
Arizona	Louisiana	New Jersey
California*	Maryland**	New York*
Florida	Massachusetts	South Carolina
Georgia	Missouri	Wisconsin

Seven states have APN title protection, but the scope of practice is authorized by both the state Board of Nursing and the state Board of Medicine. The seven states are listed below. Asterisk (*) indicates that CNSs are not included.

Idaho*	North Carolina*	South Dakota
Mississippi*	Pennsylvania*	Virginia
Nebraska*		

Four states do not provide APN title protection; APNs function under a broad nurse practice act. These states are Illinois,* Minnesota,** Ohio,* and Tennessee. Asterisk (*) indicates that CNSs are not included; double asterisks (**) indicate that only psychiatric/mental health CNSs are included.

Thirty-nine states and the District of Columbia have laws or statutes that include CNSs in the APN category and are listed below. Asterisk (*) indicates that only psychiatric/mental health CNSs are included.

Alabama	Kentucky	North Dakota
Alaska	Louisiana	Oklahoma
Arizona	Maine	South Carolina
Arkansas	Maryland*	South Dakota
Colorado	Massachusetts*	Tennessee
Connecticut	Michigan	Texas
Delaware	Minnesota*	Utah
District of Columbia	Missouri	Vermont
Florida*	Montana	Virginia
Georgia*	Nevada*	Washington
Hawaii	New Hampshire*	West Virginia
Indiana	New Jersey	Wisconsin
Iowa	New Mexico	Wyoming
Kansas		

PRESCRIPTIVE AUTHORITY

Fourteen states and the District of Columbia have laws that permit NPs to prescribe drugs, including controlled substances, independent of physician involvement in prescribing.

Alaska	Iowa	Oregon
Arizona	Maine	Vermont
Colorado	Montana	Washington (schedule V)
Delaware	New Hampshire	Wisconsin
District of Columbia	New Mexico	Wyoming

Nineteen states allow NPs to prescribe drugs (including controlled substances) with some degree of physician involvement or delegation of prescription writing. Asterisk (*) indicates that prescribing may be carried out only in narrowly specified situations.

Arkansas	Minnesota	Pennsylvania
Connecticut	Mississippi*	Rhode Island
Georgia	Nebraska	South Carolina*
Indiana	New York	South Dakota
Louisiana*	North Carolina	Utah
Maryland	North Dakota	West Virginia
Massachusetts		

Fifteen states provide legal sanctions to NPs to prescribe drugs (excluding controlled substances) with some degree of physician involvement or delegation of prescription writing. Asterisk (*) indicates that prescribing may be carried out only in narrowly specified situations.

Alabama	Kansas	New Jersey
California	Kentucky	Ohio*
Florida	Michigan	Tennessee
Hawaii	Missouri	Texas
Idaho	Nevada	Virginia

Twelve states allow NPs to dispense but not prescribe drugs. Asterisk (*) indicates that NPs may dispense drugs only in narrowly specified situations.

Alaska	Maine	New Hampshire
Arizona	Maryland	Texas*
Colorado	Missouri	Wisconsin
Delaware	Nevada	

Two states have no statutes for NP prescribing or dispensing drugs: Illinois and Oklahoma.

Every year, changes occur in state legislation regarding legal authority, prescriptive authority, and reimbursement policies. In 1994, 12 states either added independent prescriptive authority for APNs where none had existed previously or passed less restrictive legislative statutes regarding scope of practice, prescriptive authority, and reimbursement. Nurses, especially APNs, need to keep abreast of the changing legislative and political scenes and become more knowledgeable about how to respond to and affect legislation in their state. There is considerable evidence that restrictions on practice are decreasing, mainly because APNs have shown that their work is cost effective, that they adhere to guidelines and protocols in practice, and they do not overprescribe. In fact, most studies show that APNs prescribe fewer drugs than do physicians, with patient outcomes equal to those of physicians.

REFERENCES

1. Pearson LJ. Annual update of how each state stands on legislative issues affecting APN practice, *Nurse Practitioner* 20(1):13–51, 1995.
2. Pearson LJ. Annual update of how each state stands on legislative issues affecting advanced nursing practice. *Nurse Practitioner* 21(1):10–70, 1996.

BIBLIOGRAPHY

Barer ML, Evans RG, Holt M, Morrison JL. It ain't necessarily so: The cost implications of health care reform. *Health Aff* Fall: 88–99, 1994.
Hastings K. Health care reform: We need it but do we have the national will to shape our future? *Nurse Practitioner* 19(1):52, 1994.

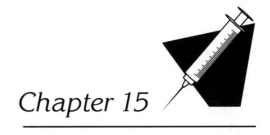

Chapter 15

Second Licensure Examination for Advanced Practice Nurses

Need for a Second Examination
Scope of the Current Examination
Responsibility for Standards
Stance of APN Professional Organizations
Summary

NEED FOR A SECOND EXAMINATION

The need for a second examination for advanced nurse practitioners (APNs) was first proposed in 1994 by the National Council of State Boards of Nursing (NCSBN) at its annual meeting. The issue is currently under discussion between the NCSBN and representatives of professional advanced practice nurses' (APNs) organizations.

The NCSBN raised the issue because of questions about APN education, standardization of educational programs, certification, and related areas. The questions specifically focused on:

- length of educational programs for APNs
- APN faculty credentials
- type and number of hours of clinical experiences
- process used to develop current certifying examinations
- frequency of recertification
- continuing education requirements
- level of current certifying examinations as to entry level requirements or higher
- qualifications required to sit for the APN examinations
- educational standards among all programs

An NCSBN task force has made known the core competencies that would be used as the basis for the new "generic" nurse practitioner (NP) examination. In March 1996, the NCSBN released a request for proposals (RFP) to perform a job analysis for NP practice, to analyze core and specialty NP activities, and to draft proposed test content. The RFP indicated that a second phase to develop a full test plan was being considered. The NCSBN indicated that it had proceeded with the RFP because it wanted to be prepared to proceed with test development, should their House of Delegates vote to do so.

In response, APN organizational representatives have pointed out that many of the competencies reflect the functions, capabilities, and professional activities of newly graduated baccalaureate nurses, not APNs, and that the proposed examination tests only very general levels of knowledge and does not address the specialized content necessary for specialized APNs. Furthermore, the answers to the questions posed at the 1994 NCSBN meeting are readily available from the American Nurses Credentialing Center (ANCC) and the American Academy of Nurse Practitioners (AANP), and two other organizations that offer certification examinations. Qualifications required to take the examinations are clearly listed, as is content covered in the examinations.

SCOPE OF THE CURRENT EXAMINATION

All APN educational programs—NP, nurse-midwifery (CNMW), clinical specialist (CNS), and nurse anesthesia (CRNA)—have been developed under rigid requirements by the appropriate specialty groups aware of the need for the highest standards of educational and clinical preparation required for practice in these areas. Most programs are part of master's degree programs in universities. The universities are accredited by the appropriate regional accrediting body; the nursing programs are accredited by both the university-accrediting body and by the National League for Nursing (NLN); the APN programs are accredited by the NLN and are operated under the educational and practice standards developed by the respective professional groups—the National Organization of Nurse Practitioner Faculties (NONPF), the American Association of Nurse Practitioners (AANP), the National Certification Corporation for the Obstetric, Gynecologic, and Neonatal Nurse Specialties (NCC), and the National Council Board of Pediatric Nurses and Pediatric Nurse Practitioners (NCBPN/P).

Most educational programs are based on NONPF's *Guidelines for Nurse Practitioner Education and Curriculum,* revised in 1995 to reflect more specific and more rigorous guidelines. Most programs have about the same credit and course requirements and clinical practice hours under a preceptor (although there are differences among the programs because of the types of clinical experiences available to students), the same extent of experience for APN faculty and preceptors, similar admission standards, and similar other variables, most of which exist because of differences among the persons involved in teaching and precepting.

The certifying examinations offered currently through ANCC and other certifying organizations are specific to each specialty and test the theoretical and clinical knowledge of the examinee. The ANCC requires the master's degree for applicants. The American College of Nurse-Midwives (ACNM) also has high standards, both for the required core competencies and the national certifying examination, which all NMWs must take to be able to practice.

RESPONSIBILITY FOR STANDARDS

Traditionally, state boards of nursing are responsible for supporting standards of practice and for registering and issuing licenses to qualified persons to practice as registered nurses or as licensed practical nurses. The education, evaluation of students, accreditation, credentialing, and all other aspects of preparing and periodically testing and recertifying nurses are the responsibility of appropriate, qualified professional groups and organizations. In light of these traditional responsibilities, the AACC, AANP, NCC, and NCBPN/P have met with the NCSBN to clarify the NCSBN's rationale for creating and requiring a generic NP examination, rather than accepting the validity and reliability of the specialty certifying examinations now offered by APN professional organizations.

STANCE OF APN PROFESSIONAL ORGANIZATIONS

At this time, the professional organizations are negotiating with the NCSBN, and NONPF has sent representatives to the NCSBN House of Delegates meeting (August 1996) to ensure the accuracy and adequacy of the NP job analysis being implemented by the NCSBN. Because the NCSBN has proceeded with plans for test development without any resolution or consensus involving the APN professional organizations, the professional certifying groups question whether NCSBN is operating in good faith.*

Last-minute update: "After lengthy negotiations that produced a mechanism for third-party evaluation, the National Council of State Boards of Nursing (NCSBN) acknowledged in late 1996 that ANCC's current nurse practitioner certification examinations meet the goal of assuring sound professional certification that can be used for regulatory purposes with legal defensibility." (American Nurses Credentialing Center, 1996–97)

The APN professional organizations oppose the new examination on the following grounds:

It is not the legitimate responsibility of boards of nursing to be involved in the education, certification, or examination of any registered nurse or licensed practical nurse.

Requiring a generic exam for NPs is not necessary and is duplicative of certifying examinations that have been in place for many years and that have been periodically updated to incorporate additional material such as health policy, case management, social and economic policy, and care of culturally diverse populations.

The proposed NCSBN examination is not as rigorous as the ANCC examinations that are specific for each specialty; because of the lower level of knowledge tested, if the NCSBN examination were used to certify APNs to practice, the standards for practicing could decrease.

NONPF's position, stated in a letter to members on July 5, 1996, is that

We are firmly committed to the position that the profession must be credentialed by the professional groups, and that the appropriate test of advanced practice nurse practitioners is measured through a specialty rather than a generic NP exam.

SUMMARY

The discussion continues between the NCSBN and APN professional organizational representatives. The goal of each group is to ensure the highest possible educational and testing standards for APNs. A generic APN examination would be very unlikely to test the knowledge and skills of the various specialty areas. The most likely resolution to the issue is to standardize APN curriculums and require the same content, including clinical reasoning using case studies, clinical skills, and scores on ANCC certification examinations.

BIBLIOGRAPHY

American Nurses Credentialing Center. NCSEN recognizes NP certification; role study to follow. *Credentialing News, Winter,* 1, 1996–97. Washington DC: American Nurses Credentialing Center.

Hahn M. Issues in nurse practitioner education: What's ahead in 1996. *Advances for Nurse Practitioners* 4(1):45–46, 58, 1996.

NCSBN task force to recommend second licensure exam for NPs. *NPNews*, 3(5):2, 7, 1995.

National Organization of Nurse Practitioner Faculties. Letter to members. July 5, 1996.

National Organization of Nurse Practitioner Faculties. *Guidelines for Nurse Practitioner Education and Curriculum*, Washington, DC: National Organization of Nurse Practitioner Faculties, 1995.

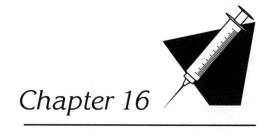

Chapter 16

Faculty Training and Faculty Practice Trends

Because of the proliferation of advanced practice nursing programs, the demand for doctorally prepared, certified advanced practice nurses (APNs) is growing at a tremendous rate. Many schools of nursing are limiting their master's degree programs to APN programs only. An added part of these programs is emphasis on preparing family nurse practitioners (FNPs) because of the demand for their services—FNPs are prepared to care for people of all ages, including babies and children, and are thus ideal for inner-city and rural practices. However, it takes more time and more clinical practice hours to educate FNPs since they must know how to diagnose and treat diseases and conditions in persons of all ages and know developmental stages of all age groups.

FACULTY TRAINING

To respond to the increasing demand and to make themselves more marketable, many doctorally prepared faculty are enrolling in post-master's APN programs. Similarly, master's prepared CNSs also see the need to add NP knowledge and skills to their repertoire of clinical expertise to enable them to retain or secure faculty positions in what now appears to be "the only game in town"—APN education and practice.

In the fall of 1995, the University of Pennsylvania School of Nursing was the first school to offer a program for APN faculty, including faculty for nurse-midwives (NMWs), to prepare these faculty to teach students in the specialty areas. The program, called the Regional Training Program for Nurse-Midwifery and Nurse Practitioner Faculty, is designed not only to enhance the didactic and clinical teaching skills of NMW and NP faculty, but to increase the number and expertise of these much needed faculty.

FACULTY PRACTICE

During the 1960s and 1970s, when schools of nursing were becoming integrated into colleges and universities with a consequent emphasis on theory, many nursing faculty did not practice and did not see the need to practice on a regular basis. However, by the early 1980s, it became evident that faculty were losing touch with the real world of patients and patient care; their detachment and decreased knowledge base were evident to students and caused faculty to lose credibility with their peers and with students. Although faculty for APN programs had generally maintained practice time despite their academic schedules, non-APN nursing faculty often had not, but they too recognized the need to remain current and to retain their clinical expertise. Therefore, although APN faculty may have led the way in many schools, all nursing faculty agreed that faculty for a practice profession must also practice; to do this they must be involved in patient care, preferably in a group practice with physicians and other APN practitioners.

Definition and Expectations of Faculty Practice

Nursing faculty have developed several definitions of faculty practice during the past 10 years; from these, a working definition currently accepted by the National Organization of Nurse Practitioner Faculties (NONPF) Faculty Practice Committee is: "Faculty practice includes all aspects of the delivery of nursing service through the roles of clinician, educator, researcher, consultant and administrator."[1] If supervision and "moonlighting" practice are considered, 90% of NP faculty members engage in practice activities.[1]

However, many schools of nursing now require that *all* nursing faculty dedicate at least one half-day per week to clinical practice; time spent supervising students in clinical training does not fulfill the requirement. Most (probably all) schools that have APN programs require that APN faculty practice at least one-half day per week. (Ideally, practice time should be at least one full day.) In addition, faculty are expected to teach, which involves continually updating lectures and clinical conference materials because of new information, procedures, and treatments that appear on the market; to mentor other faculty and involve preceptors in program activities; to conduct clinical research and write grant applications to seek support for their research; and to publish at least two articles a year in refereed journals. Most nursing faculty spend at least 80 hours a week keeping up with immediate responsibilities. Nevertheless, in the academic setting, faculty practice brings benefits in having access to patients for research, in developing current and relevant curriculum content, and in generating ideas for research and publications.

Many faculty cite disadvantages to faculty practice, such as lack of time and support from administration and few academic or monetary rewards. The latter disadvantage is almost universal, since faculty practice does not earn "points" toward tenure or promotion in most schools of nursing. Faculty who have family responsibilities must further divide what little time is left to maintain relationships and a balanced life.

Models of Faculty Practice

Many hospital departments of nursing have developed nursing practice models, several of which focus on collaborative and interdisciplinary practice. In 1993, NONPF published four models of faculty practice in various schools of nursing. The four models are the unification model, the collaborative model, the integrated model, and the entrepreneurial model.

Unification Model

The unification model unifies administrators in clinical agencies and in schools of nursing with all faculty in positions as clinicians and educators. The model, first used in 1972, was used by both Rush-Presbyterian-St. Luke's Medical Center (Chicago, IL) and the University of Rochester (NY). In 1985, Dr. Claire Fagin, dean of the school of nursing at the University of Pennsylvania, said of this faculty practice model: "These institutions [and Case Western Reserve University] raised the visibility of professional nursing practice, gave legitimacy to faculty practice, demonstrated the possibilities of autonomy for nurses and for collaborative practice with physicians and others, and won the support of powerful advocates on the national scene."[1]

Collaborative Model

The collaborative model formalizes linkages between faculty and clinicians by awarding joint appointments whereby faculty members' primary responsibilities are in the school of nursing, but they also hold appoint-

ment in a particular clinical agency, usually with salary costs shared pro-
portionately according to time and responsibilities in each setting. This
type of model is used at Case Western Reserve University and is exemplary
regarding joint appointments between schools of nursing and clinical
agencies.

Integrated Model

The integrated model, developed at Pennsylvania State University and the
University of Wisconsin at Milwaukee, allows faculty and graduate students to share responsibilities for patient care.

Entrepreneurial Model

The entrepreneurial model provides faculty the opportunity to design
their own practices, to develop practice goals and objectives, and to care
for patients as part of their faculty responsibilities. The type of practice can
involve any kind of practice setting, including private practice, inside or
outside the university. For example, some faculty elect to negotiate and
contract for a faculty practice position in an employee health service operated by the university. In all settings, faculty negotiate to be allowed to use
the setting as a teaching and research site. A salary may or may not be part
of the contract. This model provides the most flexibility for organizing
time commitment, scope of responsibilities and practice, educational activities, consulting activities, and patient-care activities.

The entrepreneurial model has been widely instituted at the University of Tennessee College of Nursing in Memphis—all faculty, including
the dean, are encouraged to develop a faculty practice. One practice site is
the Memphis Jewish Home; the nursing faculty provide primary care and
screening to residents. A contract is signed each year between the school
and the nursing home. The nursing home pays the college of nursing on a
per capita basis for services rendered. Faculty at the college also operate
the student health service. Students pay an annual fee at the time of registration and receive all primary care from nursing faculty. The college administers the program by transfer voucher for payment. The college has
subsequently expanded the arrangement by contracting with other
schools of nursing to provide primary care to students.

Evaluation of Faculty Practice Models

Evaluation of faculty practice models was designed on three parameters: degree of faculty role integration, degree of nursing control over the

practice, and degree of financial autonomy attained. The ideal model is to have the three factors equally attained. Most models do not succeed in having each part equal to the others.

INITIATING FACULTY PRACTICE

Planning

Developing a faculty practice plan is generally the first step in the process of starting a faculty practice. Similar to a business plan, the faculty practice plan outlines the organizational structure within which faculty may receive compensation for their services. Included are the bylaws, policies, and procedures that govern professional practice within the institution or school of nursing. As in academic medical centers, the institution and the school jointly develop a practice plan that enables both to understand the shared governance, costs, and revenues derived from the practice. The faculty practice plan addresses the amount of time that a faculty member may devote to practice and how much income faculty members may generate in relation to their academic salaries. The practice plan must adhere to university or institutional guidelines.

The components of the faculty practice plan should incorporate several steps:

1. Perform a comprehensive self-assessment to determine the advantages and disadvantages of beginning a faculty practice, addressing issues such as rationale, selection of faculty to be involved, the real and estimated financial resources available, how much can be dedicated to the development of the faculty practice, and the importance of a faculty practice to the school.

2. Formulate clear, concise goals (e.g., start a faculty-managed independent primary care clinic).

3. Set specific objectives, preferably with timelines (e.g., by the end of the first year of operation, the clinic will have 250 disadvantaged families enrolled).

4. Conduct a feasibility study to determine whether the practice can be successful from all perspectives.

5. Construct a business plan with the following components: marketing plan, financial plan, business review, organization and personnel, and timeline.

6. Prepare a report (usually termed an executive summary) giving precise pertinent information about the faculty practice for top-level administrators and potential financial supporters.

Setting Goals

Goals for a faculty practice plan should incorporate the rationale for the plan, the approach(es) to be taken, and the benefits of the plan. The example below is drawn from the Johns Hopkins University School of Nursing Plan.[2]

Faculty within the faculty practice plan will:

1. Provide expert clinical nursing care and stand as an outstanding example to students and faculty within the health-care system, and to the community at large.
2. Utilize a continuous quality-improvement approach and the latest research findings and standards of practice to provide the delivery of health care to individuals and communities served.
3. Demonstrate innovative approaches to the delivery of health care through the development of new practice roles for nursing, expansion of nursing practice into unique settings and partnerships, and creation of new practice models.
4. Provide opportunities for students to integrate knowledge and skills in a wide variety of clinical settings under direct faculty supervision.
5. Provide new opportunities for expansion and development of the programs of research and scholarship of the faculty and the students.
6. Provide for financial stability of programs of education, research, scholarship, and service.
7. Provide financial support for development of faculty research programs and scholarly programs, including activity supporting faculty development in these realms.
8. Provide financial support for development of faculty clinical practice and of faculty clinicians.

BARRIERS TO FACULTY PRACTICE

Administrative opposition is the most common barrier to developing a faculty practice plan within an institution. For example, in a Georgia college the dean of the school of nursing sought the university president's approval for an independent corporation, similar to that for existing medical practice groups. The dean was met with delays, canceled meetings, fault finding, misinformation, and, finally, outright refusal. Only after a business structure was created that did not require the approval of the university president was a successful faculty practice plan launched. This process was judged, in the end, to have been preferable because the slow, sure process enabled the practice to grow incrementally and successfully.

CAUSES OF FAILURE FOR FACULTY PRACTICE

Many faculty private practices have been developed, and many have failed, usually, as in any other business venture, because of

- lack of commitment of those involved
- insufficient resources
- lack of financial and legal experts to provide consultation and assistance
- underestimation of the costs and resources needed to start and operate a practice
- internal factors, such as turf battles, individual greed, battle for power and dominance, and general dissatisfaction between or among personnel
- external factors, such as decrease in number of patients to be served; increase in cost of liability insurance, increase in costs for property rental fees, insurance, or taxes; increase in competition for patients; increase in operational costs (e.g., utilities, equipment repair and replacement)

It is better to think about the disadvantages as well as the advantages when planning a faculty (or other) practice. Disadvantages occur among groups of physicians, too; they are not immune to the forces that impinge on the success of a business cooperative. Generally, planning should "start low and go slow" (a maxim applied to pharmacologic therapy of older persons) and work slowly and carefully toward expansion. Relying on outside funding is not feasible in the current economic environment; sources often seem to evaporate when they are most needed.

TRENDS IN FACULTY PRACTICE

In the past, it was customary for faculty to devote their time gratis to agencies, more or less in exchange for having students in the setting. More and more, as faculty become involved in practice, schools of nursing are negotiating to create revenue-generating or revenue-sharing faculty practices; thus, faculty no longer give away their time, and the school receives compensation for faculty time and expertise. This kind of arrangement is more realistic and necessary in this time of rapidly decreasing economic resources.

The University of California at San Francisco School of Nursing successfully changed a volunteer young women's clinic, which faculty had operated since the 1970s, into a revenue-sharing practice. Most negotiations revolved around financial issues. The experience showed that careful negotiations where mutual concerns are addressed can result in a satisfactory arrangement. The personal and professional satisfaction of having a faculty practice can be highly gratifying and can provide the impetus for continuing commitment and stability of the practice.

REFERENCES

1. National Organization of Nurse Practitioner Faculties. *Faculty Practice Models.* Washington, DC: National Organization of Nurse Practitioner Faculties, 1993.
2. John Hopkins University School of Nursing. Faculty Practice Plan, 1996 (unpublished).

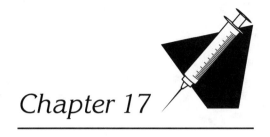

Chapter 17

Effectiveness of Advanced Practice Nurses

Advanced practice nursing has definitely "arrived"; it is now firmly established in academic settings and its graduates are much in demand by health-care facilities and consumers. Advanced practice nurses (APNs) have proven their worth in many ways and have become an integral part of health-care delivery, particularly to underserved populations. The effectiveness of nurse practitioners (NPs) and certified nurse-midwives (CNMs), in particular, has been studied for 30 years or longer. A large quantity of data show that both groups of APNs are highly effective.

NP and CNM roles evolved in response to the lack of basic services in certain parts of the country, particularly in rural and inner-city areas. The establishment of the Frontier Nursing Service in 1925 in rural Kentucky and the first NP program (a pediatric NP program) in 1965 in Colorado came about because health care was not available to large segments of the population in these areas, and physicians had chosen not to practice among the rural and inner-city poor. Today, NPs and CNMs have increased access to basic health services in a wide variety of geographic and practice settings; in many rural and inner-city areas, they are the only providers available. These nurse groups have also demonstrated their ability to enhance the delivery of care in school-based clinics, long-term care facilities and nursing homes, correctional institutions, industrial health centers, community health clinics, and birthing centers.

ASSESSMENT OF CARE

A seminal article by Barbara J. Safriet, Associate Dean of the Yale Law School, appeared in the *Yale Journal on Regulation* in 1992; the impact of her article throughout the health-care system has been unparalleled. Dr. Safriet analyzed most previous studies done on the effectiveness of NPs and CNMs, and she presented strong, objective evidence to support the effectiveness of the practices of these groups of nurses.[1]

To assess the effectiveness of a health-care provider, as Safriet points out, one must, at minimum, determine the provider's ability to deliver quality care at a reasonable cost to a significant portion of the general population or particular groups. Safriet states that these criteria have only recently been applied in a systematic way to care provided by physicians, but NPs and CNMs have been the specific focus of hundreds of effectiveness studies for more than two decades, and the results have repeatedly demonstrated superior performance of NPs and CNMs with respect to each criterion: quality, access, and cost.[1]

Quality

The most comprehensive study was released in 1986 by the Office of Technology Assessment (OTA) of the federal government, in response to a request from the Senate Committee on Appropriations, to justify federal funds allocated each fiscal year to support nursing education programs. The OTA report presented the results of an in-depth assessment of NPs, CNMs, and physician assistants (PAs) and their contribution and cost-effectiveness in meeting health-care needs in the United States. Analysis of the numerous studies that had assessed the quality of care, encompassing both technical care and the art of care (humanitarian aspects), led the OTA to conclude that "within their areas of competence, NPs and CNMs provide care whose quality is equivalent to that of care provided by physicians."[2] This conclusion provided the rationale needed to justify the appropriation of federal monies to support nursing education programs, whose graduates contribute significantly to meeting the nation's health-care needs.

The studies analyzed process measures (using the factors of adequacy of pediatric assessment, adequacy of prescribing medications, and the degree of short- and long-term patient compliance) and outcome measures (resolution of acute problems, improvement in patients' physical, emotional, and social functional status, and reduction in pain or discomfort among pediatric populations). Other studies demonstrated a difference in the quality of care of NPs and physicians—in 12 of 14 studies, the relative quality of care given by NPs was better than that given by physicians. In these studies, the process measures included number of diagnostic tests, effectiveness of interpersonal management, and thoroughness of diagnosis and treatment documentation; the outcome measures were blood pressure control in patients with hypertension, the degree of weight reduction in obese patients, reduction of pain or discomfort in adult patients, and level of activity limitation and anxiety in patients with chronic health problems. Physicians were judged better at managing problems that required technical solutions, a finding that reflects the fact that physicians receive much more extensive technical training than do NPs and CNMs.

The OTA study found equally positive conclusions about the quality of care provided by CNMs, and stated that CNMs "can manage normal pregnancies safely, and can manage these patients as well as, or better, than physicians." Mortality (fetal, perinatal, neonatal, and maternal) was the same for care by physicians and by CNMs.[2]

Safriet found that

> the quality of care by NPs and CNMs is crucially important for two reasons: first, their effective deployment depends on their ability to render care that is safe and effective, and, second, the most frequently articulated basis for physicians' opposition to these and other non-physician providers has been concern about their ability to provide high-quality care.[1]

Thus, the OTA study, and others, have shown that the care provided by NPs and CNMs is equivalent to care provided by physicians for comparable services.

Satisfaction

Patient satisfaction was a part of the OTA analyses; the conclusion was that patients were very satisfied with the care provided by NPs. Supportive evidence for the conclusion was that successful malpractice cases against NPs are extremely rare.

A study of physicians' satisfaction with NP performance showed that a major factor in establishing collegial relationships between NPs and physicians is the length of time and proximity between physicians and NPs in practice settings; physicians who had worked closely with NPs over longer periods of time became more satisfied with the quality of care provided by NPs.[3]

PREVENTIVE CARE

In the past 10 years in the United States, greater emphasis has been placed on preventing illness and disease by changing lifestyles and promoting health through education and self-care—people have begun taking more responsibility for their own health. NPs and CNMs have been particularly effective in this area because of their focus on patient education, continuity of care over time, and holistic approach to providing care by taking into account not only their patients' physical status, but their psychological, social, and financial status, and their family and community support systems.

All nurses prepared at the bachelor's degree level have coursework, both theory and clinical practice, in community health, epidemiology, demographics, and statistics. The preparation assists them to collect, analyze, and interpret data about large groups of people. This knowledge, added to the advanced education and expert skills acquired at the master's degree level, allows NPs and CNMs to provide comprehensive care to all ages in all settings.

APNs also keep abreast of emerging trends, government recommendations, and current research about illness, disease, epidemics, emerging infectious diseases, immunization schedules, and appropriate screening tests to detect diseases in their early stages. Information of this nature is compiled by the U.S. Preventive Services Task Force.[4] Another valuable source of health and prevention information is *Healthy People 2000,* a 1992 publication compiled by agencies within the U.S. Department of Health and Human Services.[5] The agencies developed comprehensive objectives regarding the health status of the U.S. population to be achieved in the coming decade. Issues such as demographics, prevalence and incidence of specific diseases, health promotion, health protection, preventive services, and disease surveillance are discussed in detail. Objectives relate specifically to all age groups, particularly to low-income and minority groups. This publication is especially significant for providers of primary care. Knowing what the national objectives are and the focus of objectives and special health-care needs, especially of minority and underserved populations, helps guide APN practice and patient education.

FEDERAL SUPPORT

Federal funds to support health professionals' education programs have been available since 1963, when the Health Professions Educational Assistance Act was passed, authorizing $175 million for the construction of training facilities for physicians, dentists, nurses, and other health professionals.[6] This law was the first successful legislation against the long-held majority opposition to federal assistance for health education, and it formed the basis for the Nurse Training Act of 1964.[7]

Federal support of NP and CNM programs has been the single greatest impetus for the development and growth of these programs for the past 32 years. Securing federal support indicates that recipients meet criteria of significance, demand, quality, and capability. Federal funds have been appropriated for nursing education programs through the Division of Nursing, first to the Special Projects Program, then the Advanced Nursing Education Program to increase the number of master's and doctorally prepared nurses, and finally, to the Nurse Practitioner and Nurse-Midwifery Program, which has received an average of $11.5 million each fiscal year since 1975. That level of funding remained almost constant, gradually increasing to $14.7 million in 1992. Appropriations for fiscal year 1997 to the Division of Nursing, Bureau of Health Professions, Human Resources and Services Administration, Department of Health and Human Services are expected to be about $16 million for the Nurse Practitioner and Nurse-Midwifery Grant program. In addition, the following funding is expected*:

Advanced Education	$11,176,000
Nurse Anesthetist	$ 2,471,000
Special Projects	$ 9,454,000
Diversity (Minorities) Program	$ 3,462,000
Professional Nurse Traineeships	$14,237,000

SUMMARY

APNs have established a reputation for delivering outstanding care, are recognized for their capabilities and expertise, and are now in greater demand than ever before in all settings. Representatives of major foundations state unequivocally that public health nurses, prepared as APNs, are needed to provide care to underinsured and underserved populations, particularly among diverse cultural groups. Many nurse educators advocate that part of the basic education of future APNs include public health nursing. Many programs already have public health nursing as a foundation for APN education. The explosive growth and development of technology and information systems and new research findings showing the impact of genetics on a person's health also have vast implications for the training and practice of APNs.

---

*Source: Captain Thomas P. Phillips, PhD, RN, and Chief, Nursing Education, Division of Nursing (November 25, 1996, telephone communication).

In addition, APNs must know legislative processes and how public policy is changed or mandated with regard to health care. The art and science of negotiation is necessary in today's world. APNs need to know organizations and how they operate. Patients in the future will act more independently and responsibly in caring for themselves and will require greater knowledge about their particular health problems, medications, treatments, and immediate and long-term needs. At the same time, health professionals must interact continuously with community organizations and groups to promote the health of entire neighborhoods, not just individuals within the community.

All these areas require more cost-effective, creative, and efficient methods to educate nurses now and for the future. Changes in perceptions, biases, and level of involvement must occur. Using past accomplishments as a base, nurses will be able to realize their highest potential.

REFERENCES

1. Safriet BJ. Health care dollars and regulatory sense: The role of advanced practice nursing. *Yale J Regulation*, 9(2):417–488, 1992.
2. Office of Technology Assessment. *Nurse Practitioners, Physician Assistants, and Certified Nurse-Midwives: A Policy Analysis*. Washington, DC: Office of Technology Assessment, 1986.
3. Hanson CE. Nominations for excellence: Collegial advocacy for nurse practitioners. *J Am Acad Nurse Pract* 6(10):471–476, 1994.
4. U.S. Preventive Services Task Force. *Guide to Clinical Preventive Services*, 2nd ed. Alexandria, VA: International Medical Publishing, 1996.
5. U.S. Department of Health and Human Services, Public Health Service. *Healthy People 2000: National Health Promotion and Disease Prevention Objectives*. Boston: Jones and Bartlett, 1992.
6. U.S. Congress, Senate, Committee on Labor and Public Welfare. *Health Professions Educational Assistance Act of 1963* (H.R. 12, H.R. 109), 88th Congress. Washington, DC: U.S. Government Printing Office, 1980.
7. U.S. Public Health Service, Bureau of Health Manpower Education, Division of Nursing. *Nurse Training Act: Title VIII—Public Health Service Act, the Complete Law:* National Training Act of 1964 (P.L. 85-581), National Training Act of 1971 (P.L. 92-158). Washington, DC: U.S. Government Printing Office, 1972.

BIBLIOGRAPHY

Davis AR. The division of nursing and its relationship to nurse practitioner education. *J Am Acad Nurse Pract* 4(4):162–165, 1992.

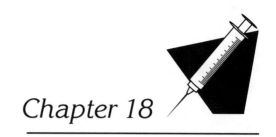

Chapter 18

Epilogue

A Personal Note on Physicians and Nurses

During my own experiences as a nurse for 50 years and as a nurse practitioner for almost 20 years, I have encountered only a very few physicians with whom I would not care to work under any circumstances. In nearly all my encounters with physicians and surgeons, I have found them to be professional, courteous, highly skilled, knowledgeable, and willing (often eager) to answer questions or clarify any area of written or verbal orders, patient care (including estimated progress/prognosis), extended plans of care, responses to medications or treatments, and so forth.

For example, my first clinical rotation as a "probie" (probationer) nursing student at Kings County Hospital, Brooklyn, New York, in 1946, was in the cancer building. At that time, only terminal cancer patients were cared for because at that time diagnosis was usually not made until the disease was far advanced. Treatment was primarily radical surgery and radiation therapy; the chemotherapeutic drugs had not yet been developed. Dr. Joseph Cresci was then the chief resident. He was a born teacher, and he taught both medical and nursing students more than we would have learned from others about all kinds of patient problems and whether they related to cancer care and treatment. Dr. Cresci always gathered any of us who were free to see procedures, to attend patient rounds, to observe wound debridement and dressing, or to hear about particular signs and symptoms exhibited by patients. I particularly remember his pointing out to us the typical dermatological sign of extensive breast cancer known as "peau d'orange," which is rarely seen today. Coincidentally, I am currently working with Dr. Cresci's daughter-in-law, who corroborates my perception that he was a truly exceptional teacher, by telling me that, even in his eighties, medical students transported him to a classroom or gathering place so that he could tutor them to pass the medical board examinations to become licensed as physicians. He practiced in Brooklyn for over 50 years and was beloved by all who knew him.

I remember many such physicians and surgeons, not all by name, but their faces are as clear to me now as they were years ago. In particular, and in addition to Dr. Cresci, were Drs. Hector Benoit, Bernard Ficarra, George Magovern, Nelson Holden, Louis Helman, Norman Meyer, William Druckemiller, Robert Bell, John O'Brien, John Harley, Edmund Dombrowski, Harry Kaplan, John Malfetano, Frank Cifarelli, Victor Dembrow, James Fontana, Max Berliner, Joseph McGoldrick, Benjamin Woodword, and James Gittings. These doctors worked long hours, for little salary, and were dedicated and committed to their patients. That year of internship was especially grueling, with 20-hour days and nights, on-call status, and hours of holding retractors in the operating room. The physicians and surgeons taught me a great deal. Not only do I admire and respect them, but I am considerably in their debt for enthusiastically conveying that medicine and learning are both exciting and challenging. Most of these physicians have probably retired or have died—losses to the medical and surgical communities.

However, I cannot say that all physicians were courteous, interested in teaching, and uniformly kind to nurses—students or otherwise. Many were sarcastic, intimidating, even abusive. But they were the exceptions.

Today, more than ever, professional multidisciplinary health-care teams provide the best care, at the lowest cost, particularly when physicians and nurse practitioners work together collaboratively, with mutual respect and trust, each acknowledging the strengths of the other.

Appendices

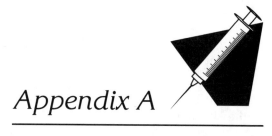

Appendix A

Clinical Reasoning

Thinking, decision making, and clinical reasoning are components of the process of correlating all objective and subjective information that is available in a given situation, about one person or a group, to arrive at accurate assessment and valid conclusions which lead a person to make final decisions and to act appropriately.

How people think is a highly individual matter, depending on the individual's genetic makeup, past experiences, and ability to take in and process information as quickly as possible, then to act or at least to correctly assess and interpret the status of the person or thing (environment) being examined. The following sections describe some components that enter into the process of thinking and deciding.

Organization—one's "computer brain" automatically organizes and files all input data. It is important that a person know how his/her own mind works to organize facts. Complete understanding of organizational processes is probably not possible; however, we can pay attention to what facts are put together and in what order they are arranged.

Memory, both short-term and long-term, is a vital function of the brain. As people age, one or both types of memory become unreliable and, ultimately, totally nonfunctional. Training can improve memory—simply use memory consciously and deliberately by memorizing lists of various subjects and repeating from memory the information on the list. Memory aids are useful for most of us, regardless of age, and help us remember the most important or pertinent details.

Consistency is concerned with how well one thinks over time. Fluctuation in thinking abilities occurs frequently and is probably quite normal, depending on how we feel physically and mentally. Both internal and external factors affect how we feel—what we eat, how much sleep we have had, what the weather is, how our relationships with other people are going at any particular time. The best we can do is to know what affects our ability to think at the highest level and put into place, as much as possible, the conditions that help us to think and to remember at the maximal level.

Intuition plays a primary role in our thinking, correlating, and decision making processes. Often, we act only on intuition—what seems or "feels" right or is the best thing to do. Often, intuition is based on extensive past experience in dealing with similar situations or individuals. We may have forgotten many of our past experiences, but our subconscious retains the memories and helps us to decide and to act, almost without our being aware of our thought processes in the current situation. It is almost as if someone else makes the decision or leads us to act.

Emotions, or our psychological perspective, also enter into thinking and decision making. Our feelings sometimes influence us too much at times, and we make decisions based on the moment's anger, hurt, or frustration rather than on the specific facts that are presented to us. In certain situations, our emotions can halt our thinking processes altogether, and rational thought becomes impossible—we decide or act only on emotion. A very strong emotion such as fear can affect us in this way—the only thought becomes the urgency to survive.

CLINICAL REASONING

Kassirer and Kopelman (1991) describe in detail the various components that make up the process of clinical reasoning, the end result of which is an accurate diagnosis on which to base relevant and appropriate treatment. These components embody knowledge from cognitive science, decision theory, and computer science (artificial intelligence). Much of our knowledge in these areas is incomplete. However, in recent decades, scientists and researchers working in the field of human problem solving and human intelligence have made great strides in clarifying reasoning processes and the steps through which the reasoning person progresses to arrive at conclusions.

New Patient—First Encounter

To propel the patient along the right path regarding diagnosis and treatment, rapid, basic decisions must be made when a new patient enters the clinic or outpatient center. The algorithm presented in Figure A-A provides the initial steps in this process.

Diagnosis is a process of inference in which diagnosticians derive inferences from observation such as historical data, physical findings, and laboratory test results, all of which lead them to a "working diagnosis." The working diagnosis is an accepted basis on which to develop a plan of treatment and a prognosis. During the inferential process, the clinician uses many strategies to combine, integrate, and interpret data. These strategies include shortcuts or rules of thumb, known as *heuristics*, which incorporates accumulated knowledge and experiences from many sources by which comparisons can be made in cases that are similar or that have common characteristics. It should be pointed out to students that heuristical reasoning can result in erroneous conclusions; however, its use by experienced clinicians who have a wealth of knowledge to draw from can be highly accurate and a great time-saver. Clinicians also use established patterns for methodical collection of information, which enables them to automatically cluster related pieces of information together in "chunks" for later processing. Even the highly experienced clinician knows, however, that one should never take anything for granted without checking.

At the beginning of a patient encounter, the clinician generates preliminary diagnostic hypotheses, which can be quite broad (infection) or very specific (acute inferior myocardial infarction). Initial diagnostic hypotheses form the basis for further information gathering by pointing directions in which to go. The efficiency and speed of this process are directly related to the clinician's experience and fund of knowledge. Initially, the clinician's hypotheses are based on such routine pieces of information as age, race, sex, appearance, and chief complaint. Additional hypotheses are generated as new findings arise. The process is continually undergoing revision, with some early hypotheses being cast aside in favor of those that appear more cogent. The goal of the process of generating and revising diagnostic hypotheses is arrive at the working diagnosis. Verifying hypotheses rests on three factors: coherence, in which all pieces of data, symptoms and signs, and laboratory test results appear to make sense in their totality; adequacy, in which the clinician judges whether all pieces of information relate to all of the patient's signs and symptoms; and parsimony, which is true when all the findings lead logically to the specific diagnosis.

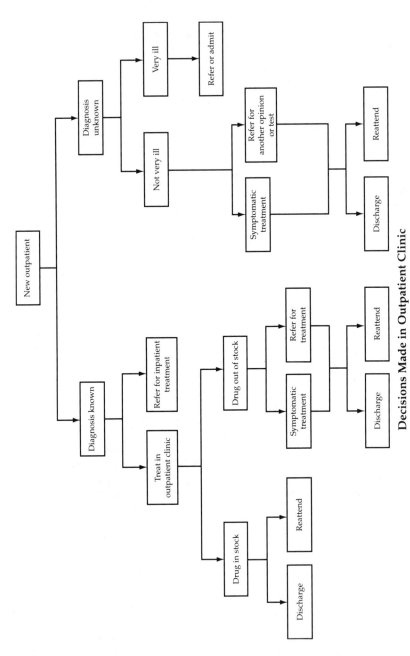

Decisions Made in Outpatient Clinic

Source: Essex BJ. *Diagnostic Pathways in Clinical Medicine: An Epidemiological Approach to Clinical Problems.* Oceanside, NY: Professional Seminar Consultants, Inc. (1981), p. 164.

When the diagnosis is established, management follows when the clinician can outline a projected clinical course, decide whether or not to order further tests, and decide on the appropriate treatment protocol to follow.

Treatment and diagnosis are intertwined, with the principles of treatment resting on the accuracy of the diagnosis. Rarely, diagnoses may be incorrect, so that a patient receives treatment for a disease that they do not have, or a patient with an (undiagnosed) disease does not receive needed treatment. With almost every treatment, there are attendant risks. For the patient without a disease who is treated, that patient receives no benefits from the treatment, yet is subject to the risks related to the treatment.

Decision thresholds come into play and occur when the clinician comes to a point where two paths are possible: treating or not treating, or treating as opposed to additional testing. The decisions in these cases rest on higher or lower probabilities in terms of the threshold for decision making. In one case, one decision is appropriate; in another, a different decision is appropriate. A decision tree is helpful, where benefits and risks are plotted for each possible action, with the weight of evidence of one or the other (benefits/risks) leading to the only right decision at that time, with that particular patient. Hindsight later may prove the decision to be incorrect, but in caring for patients, as in all other circumstances demanding decisions, one makes the best decision one can at the time, given the information then available.

Differential Diagnosis

The clinician's most critical decisions are those around making a correct diagnosis. Beginning practitioners are often perplexed and confused at the fast pace of general or family practice in which patients of all ages have complex and multiple problems that can be physical, emotional, social, environmental, or a combination of two (or more) of these components. As students, clinicians proceed in an orderly way as they collect and assess data, historical information, and physical examination findings. They can usually arrive at a correct diagnosis with careful and systematic analysis of the data. In practice, under pressure, practitioners need to focus on the patients' symptoms—their patterns and potential meanings, on characteristics of normal and abnormal human behavior, and on the effects of lifestyle and environment.

Symptoms may not be associated with any particular disease, and essential information may be lacking. What at first may seem like a physical problem may not be the real critical problem; for example, a family may no longer be able to cope with the situation in terms of stress, financial worries, or space. Seeking the answer to the question, "What made you decide to come to the clinic today?" usually elicits specific information from which to analyze the problem from the patient's perspective. Further questioning of family members can help to fill in the missing pieces.

After collecting as much information as possible from all sources—patient's history and physical examination, laboratory test results, family members—the clinician recognizes that a definitive diagnosis may not be possible at present, because of insufficient time, incomplete information, or a disease that is in process of development.

At any point in the patient encounter, the clinician makes a list of possible diagnoses, the purpose of which is not to limit the possibilities, but to include as many as possible so that no viable diagnosis is missed. When the list seems complete, the process of "ruling out" begins, aided by additional information, more laboratory tests, new symptoms, or simply time. When a diagnosis seems impossible at this time, the clinician asks that the patient return for a follow-up visit. Immediate treatment may consist of allaying fears or prescribing some type of medication that will alleviate at least some symptoms (e.g., recommending a laxative to cure an expressed problem with constipation). A telephone number is provided to the patient so that, if anything untoward occurs between this and the next visit, the patient or family can contact the practitioner. Meanwhile, the clinician reviews carefully all of the available information and recalls as much as possible of the oral communication from both patient and family, then analyzes the information again, using algorithms or other means to define and weigh the various factors involved in the patient's problem. In this process, the clinician is careful to focus on arriving at correct diagnoses and to remember that there is a 26% probability that a perfectly healthy person will have an abnormal result if six laboratory tests are done, since the norm is defined as within two standard deviations around the mean.

LIVING WITH UNCERTAINTY

In primary care practice, uncertainty is a given. The degree of uncertainty faced by primary care clinicians is greater than that encountered by other providers, because of the larger number of undifferentiated problems and relative lack of research data to help guide diagnostic reasoning. The clinician may not be able to make a diagnosis or may need to wait a period of time before the diagnosis becomes certain. Sometimes, clinicians are treating only symptoms that may resolve spontaneously before a diagnosis can be made. Diagnostic uncertainty is a result of (1) cognitive uncertainty, which is related to the practitioner's perception of the clinical problem, (2) the feeling state (usually anxiety) of the practitioner, and (3) the variability of the patient's responses to communication and treatment.

In resolving uncertainty, *time* is a powerful ally, but using time effectively takes considerable skill. The clinician who is too anxious to wait for an evolving disease to become evident may order unnecessary tests and have the patient return too frequently, at considerable cost. Conversely, the clinician who does not consider more than one hypothesis or who does not ask the patient to return could miss the diagnosis entirely. In family practice, the variety of potential decisions is much greater. Decisions may involve giving reassurance, dealing with a problem other than the presenting one, checking the patient more than once, counseling the patient and family, collecting data from many sources (family, other practitioners, psychotherapists, physical therapists, and others), initiating a clinical trial of a drug to determine its efficacy in relieving the problem, and arranging for community resources such as home care, rehabilitation, or a social worker.

Although a plethora of alternatives may be available in every situation, primary care also provides unique opportunities and positive actions: management of the presenting problem, enhancement of the clinician-patient relationship, modification of help-seeking behaviors, management of continuing problems, teaching about health promotion, enlargement of the database for individual patients, and enriching patients' knowledge about their condition and how they can participate in their own treatment.

Methods for managing uncertainty and its attendant stress include sharing feelings with colleagues and other health-care professionals, educating patients about possible outcomes, and reassuring patients that you will continue to consider all possible sources of information for diagnostic clues. Managing clinical uncertainty is an essential element to the art and science of primary care to enable the practitioner to continue to develop self-confidence and to remain functional at the optimal level. Continuous communication between practitioner and patient is critical.

BIBLIOGRAPHY

Essex BJ. *Diagnostic Pathways in Clinical Medicine: An Epidemiological Approach to Clinical Problems.* Oceanside, NY: Professional Seminar Consultants, Inc., 1981.
Kassirer JP, Kopelman RI. *Learning Clinical Reasoning.* Baltimore: Williams & Wilkins, 1991.
Rubenfeld MG, Scheffer BK. *Critical Thinking in Nursing: An Interactive Approach.* Philadelphia: Lippincott, 1995.

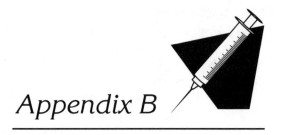

Appendix B

Maryland Nurse Practice Act for Nurse Practitioners

This appendix contains information quoted directly from Maryland State Board of Nursing.

NURSE PRACTITIONER PRACTICE

Definitions

1. "Joint Committee" means the Joint Committee on Nurse Practitioners, composed of an equal number of members appointed by the Physician Quality Assurance and Nursing Boards.
2. "Medical Board" means the Board of Physician Quality Assurance.
3. "Nursing Board" means the Board of Nursing.
4. "Nurse practitioner" means a registered nurse who by reason of certification under these regulations may engage in the activities authorized by these regulations.
5. "Personally prepare and dispense" means that a nurse practitioner:
   a. Is physically present on the premises where the prescription is filled; and
   b. Performs a final check of the prescription before the prescription is provided to the patient.
6. "Physician" means an individual licensed to practice medicine in this State.
7. "Starter dosage" means an amount of a drug sufficient to begin therapy:
   a. Of a short duration of 72 hours or less; or
   b. Before obtaining a larger quantity of the drug to complete therapy.

8. "Written agreement" means the development and implementation of a written agreement between a nurse practitioner and a licensed physician concerning the performance by the nurse practitioner of the functions authorized by these regulations.

NURSE PRACTITIONER—SCOPE AND STANDARDS OF PRACTICE

A. A nurse practitioner may perform independently the following functions under the terms and conditions set forth in the written agreement:
   1. Comprehensive physical assessment of patients;
   2. Establish medical diagnosis for common short-term or chronic stable health problems;
   3. Order, perform, and interpret laboratory tests;
   4. Prescribe drugs;
   5. Perform therapeutic or corrective measures;
   6. Refer patients to appropriate licensed physicians or other health care providers;
   7. Provide emergency care.
B. Before a nurse practitioner may practice he shall:
   1. Obtain certification under these regulations;
   2. Enter into a written agreement with a physician whereby the physician on a regularly scheduled basis shall:
      a. Accept referrals,
      b. Establish and review drug and other medical guidelines with the nurse practitioner,
      c. Participate with the nurse practitioner in periodically reviewing and discussing medical diagnoses and the therapeutic or corrective measures employed in the practice setting,
      d. Jointly sign records if needed to document accountability of both the physician and nurse practitioner,
      e. Be available for consultation in person, by telephone, or by some other form of telecommunication, and
      f. Designate an alternate physician if the physician identified in the written agreement temporarily becomes unavailable;
   3. Obtain approval of the written agreement as set forth in Regulation .06.
C. A nurse practitioner may practice only in the area of specialization in which he is certified.
D. A nurse practitioner shall immediately advise the Nursing Board if a written agreement is ended by either party.
E. A nurse practitioner shall submit a new or amended written agreement for approval before:

    1. Altering the practice setting; or

    2. Modifying or expanding the medical functions that the nurse practitioner is authorized to perform.

F. A State certified nurse practitioner who is otherwise in full compliance with these regulations and who joins a group practice of State certified nurse practitioners that has an approved written agreement on file with the Nursing Board, instead of submitting a written agreement, may submit an affidavit verifying that the nurse practitioner and a physician have discussed the written agreement and mutually agree to practice within its framework.

G. A nurse practitioner has a right and obligation to refuse to perform any delegated act, oral or written, if in the nurse practitioner's judgment, it is unsafe or an invalidly prescribed medical act.

Certification

A. An applicant for certification as a nurse practitioner shall:

    1. Hold a current license to practice registered nursing in the State;

    2. Complete in full the application for certification as a nurse practitioner for each area in which certification is sought;

    3. Pay all fees established by the Nursing Board;

    4. Complete a program for preparation of nurse practitioners approved by the Nursing Board; and

    5. Pass an examination as designated by the Nursing Board.

B. The Nursing Board shall:

    1. Maintain an up-to-date list of all nurse practitioners certified in the State; and

    2. Include on the nurse practitioner's registered nursing license an indication that the licensee is certified as a nurse practitioner and a designation of the nurse practitioner's area of specialization.

Renewal of Certification

A. A certification as a nurse practitioner expires at the same time as the nurse practitioner's registered nursing license unless the certification is renewed for a 1-year term as provided in this regulation.

B. Before a nurse practitioner's certification expires, the practitioner may renew for an additional 1-year term, if the nurse practitioner:

    1. Is otherwise entitled to be certified;

    2. Pays to the Nursing Board all appropriate renewal fees set by the Nursing Board; and

    3. Submits to the Nursing Board:

        a. A renewal application on the form that it requires, and

b. Satisfactory evidence that any certification received is current if that certificate was the basis for the certification issued under these regulations.

JOINT COMMITTEE ON NURSE PRACTITIONERS

A. The Nursing and Medical Boards shall establish a joint committee to do the following:
   1. Develop a written framework to be used in writing written agreements; and
   2. Make recommendations to the Nursing Board regarding approval of written agreements submitted for review, except that no written agreement may be approved by the Nursing Board unless the Medical Board reviews and approves the physician's role as described in the written agreement.
B. The joint committee shall be composed of an equal number of members appointed by the Nursing and Medical Boards.
C. Members of the joint committee may be members of the Nursing or Medical Boards or may be designees of each appointing Board.

UNLAWFUL PRACTICES

A. Unless authorized to practice under these regulations, an individual may not use the words "nurse practitioner" or any other words, letters, or symbols with the intent to represent that the individual is a nurse practitioner.
B. Any person certified under these regulations shall be subject to disciplinary sanctions set forth in Health Occupations Article, Annotated Code of this State.
C. Nothing in these regulations limits or prohibits a registered nurse from performing those functions which constitute the practice of registered nursing as defined by law.

PRESCRIBING AND DISPENSING

A. A nurse practitioner may personally prepare and dispense any drug that a nurse practitioner is authorized to prescribe in the course of treating a patient at:
   1. A medical facility or clinic that specializes in the treatment of medical cases reimbursable through workers' compensation insurance;

    2. A medical facility or clinic that is operated on a nonprofit basis;

    3. A health center that operates on a campus of an institution of higher education;

    4. A public health facility; a medical facility under contract with a State or local health department, or a facility funded with public funds; or

    5. A nonprofit hospital or a nonprofit hospital outpatient facility as authorized under the policies established by the hospital.

B. A nurse practitioner who personally prepares and dispenses a drug in the course of treating a patient shall:

    1. Comply with the labeling requirements of Health Occupations Article Title 8, Annotated Code of this State;

    2. Record the dispensing of the prescription drug on the patient's chart;

    3. Allow the Division of Drug Control to enter and inspect the nurse practitioner's office at all reasonable hours;

    4. Except for starter dosages or samples dispensed without charge, provide the patient with a written prescription; and

    5. Stamp all Schedule III, IV, and V prescriptions with the letter "C" in red ink, not less than 1 inch high in the lower right hand corner.

C. A nurse practitioner shall:

    1. Maintain two separate files, one for Schedule II prescriptions and another file for all other prescriptions; and

    2. Maintain all prescriptions for 5 years.

D. A nurse practitioner may personally prepare and dispense a starter dosage of any drug the nurse practitioner is authorized to prescribe. The nurse practitioner shall:

    1. Label the starter dosage in compliance with the labeling requirements of Health Occupations Article Title 8, Annotated Code of this State;

    2. Provide the starter dose free of charge; and

    3. Enter the starter dose dispensed in the patient's medical record.

BIBLIOGRAPHY

Maryland State Board of Nursing. Nurse Practice Act, Annotated Code of Maryland, Health Occupations Article, Title 8, and Code of Maryland Regulations, Title 10, Subtitle 27. Baltimore: Maryland State Board of Nursing, 1995. Used by permission.

Dorsey D, Executive Director, Maryland State Board of Nursing (September 1995, personal communication).

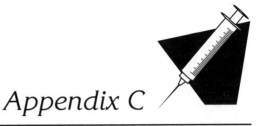

Appendix C

Maryland Nurse Practice Act and Regulations for Nurse-Midwifery

This appendix contains information quoted directly from Maryland State Board of Nursing.

Definitions

1. "ACNM" means the American College of Nurse-Midwives.
2. "ACNMCC" means the American College of Nurse-Midwives Certification Council.
3. "Board" means the Board of Nursing.
4. "BPQA" means the Board of Physician Quality Assurance.
5. "Certified nurse-midwife" means a registered nurse who is certified by the ACNM.
6. "Delegated medical functions" means those functions that come within the definition of "practice medicine" of the Health Occupations Article Section 14-101 (i), Annotated Code of Maryland, that have been delegated to a Maryland certified nurse-midwife to perform and that are specified in the written agreement.
7. "Formulary" means an approved list of the categories of substances commonly used in the practice of nurse-midwifery as determined by the Board in consultation with the Pharmacy and Medical Boards.
8. "Joint committee" means the Joint Committee on Nurse-Midwifery composed of an equal number of members appointed by the Nursing and Medical Boards.
9. "Newborn" means an infant in the first 48 hours of life.

10. "Nurse midwifery" means the health care management of newborns and clients throughout their reproductive life cycle.
11. "Pharmacy Board" means the State Board of Pharmacy.
12. "Physician" means an individual licensed to practice medicine in this State.
13. "Protocol" means a written document, approved by both the Maryland certified nurse-midwife and the physician, that details the procedures, management, and delegated medical functions that the Maryland certified nurse-midwife will follow.
14. "Written agreement" means the development and implementation of a written document between a certified nurse-midwife and a physician concerning the performance of delegated medical functions authorized by these regulations.

REQUIREMENTS FOR MARYLAND CERTIFICATION TO PRACTICE NURSE-MIDWIFERY

A. Requirements for Applicant. An applicant for Maryland certification to practice nurse-midwifery shall:
   1. Hold a current license to practice registered nursing in Maryland;
   2. Hold a current certification as a nurse-midwife from the ACNM;
   3. Complete in full the application for Maryland certification as a nurse-midwife;
   4. Have a written agreement with a physician signed by the physician and nurse-midwife which has been approved according to the requirements in Regulation .07A(2); and
   5. Pay all fees established by the Nursing Board.
B. Written Agreement
   1. The written agreement shall be on a form prescribed by the Nursing Board and the Medical Board.
   2. The nurse-midwife shall submit the written agreement to the Nursing Board.
   3. In the case of a nurse-midwife who will perform deliveries, the nurse-midwife shall have an agreement with a licensed physician who has unrestricted privileges to practice obstetrics and gynecology in a hospital in the geographic area in which the certified nurse-midwife will practice. This agreement shall be approved according to the requirements in Regulation .07A(2).
   4. In the case of a nurse-midwife who will not perform deliveries and the physician does not have privileges to practice obstetrics in a hospital in the geographic area in which the nurse-midwife will practice, the written agreement will be referred to the Joint Com-

mittee for its review and determination of whether the physician has had sufficient training and experience in obstetrics and gynecology to perform his responsibilities under the written agreement. This agreement will be approved according to the requirements in Regulation .07A(2).

5. The approved written agreement will be filed with the Nursing Board and shall be made available to the Medical Board.

6. A certified nurse-midwife who is otherwise in full compliance with these regulations and who joins a practice of certified nurse-midwives that has a written agreement with a physician on file with the Board, shall submit, on the required form, an affidavit to that effect.

7. The written agreement shall include the categories of substances selected from the approved formulary that may be prescribed and dispensed by the certified nurse-midwife.

C. Duties of the Nursing Board. The Nursing Board shall:

1. Maintain an up-to-date list of all certified nurse-midwives in this State; and

2. Include on the nurse-midwife's registered nursing license an indication that the licensee is certified as a nurse-midwife.

Practice Before State Certification

A. A registered nurse who meets the qualifications to sit for the ACNMCC national certifying examination or who has taken that examination and is waiting for the results of it may practice as a nurse-midwife graduate before certification if the:

1. Practice is under the supervision of a certified nurse-midwife who shall be physically available to the nurse-midwife graduate;

2. Supervising certified nurse-midwife agrees on a written supervision agreement on the required form to provide the supervision; and

3. Nurse-midwife graduate files with the Board a copy of the admission slip to the ACNMCC national certifying examination and a copy of the supervision agreement; there shall also be submitted to the Board on the required form an affidavit signed by the collaborating physician stating that the physician agrees to the nurse-midwife graduate's supervised practice according to the certified nurse-midwife's agreement and protocols.

B. A nurse-midwife graduate who has entered into such a supervision agreement shall immediately notify the Board, the supervising certified nurse-midwife, and the physician of the results of the ACNMCC national certifying examination.

C. A nurse-midwife graduate may not continue to practice under that supervision for more than 1 year from the filing of all documents required

under Section A, or after the denial of ACNMCC certification, whichever occurs first.

Scope of Practice

A. A Certified nurse-midwife who meets the requirements of Regulation
   .02 of this chapter may perform the following functions:
   1. Independent management of clients appropriate to the skill and
      knowledge of the certified nurse-midwife and the nurse-midwife's
      agreement and protocols;
   2. Management, in collaboration with a physician, of clients with med-
      ical complications;
   3. Referral of clients with complications beyond the scope of practice of
      the certified nurse-midwife to a licensed physician; and
   4. Consultations with and referral to other health care professionals in
      the delivery and evaluation of health care.
B. A certified nurse-midwife shall keep a record of all cases attended.
C. A certified nurse-midwife shall immediately advise the Board if the
   written agreement is ended by either party and the Board shall immediately notify the BPQA.
D. A certified nurse-midwife has the right and obligation to refuse to
   perform any delegated act, oral or written, if, in the certified nurse-midwife's judgment, it is unsafe or an invalidly prescribed medical
   act or beyond the competence of the certified nurse-midwife, in which
   case the nurse-midwife shall notify the physician at once.

Joint Committee on Nurse-Midwifery

A. The Board and the BPQA shall establish a Joint Committee to:
   1. Develop a written framework to be used in writing written
      agreements;
   2. Make recommendations to the Board regarding approval or written
      agreements submitted for review, provided, however, a written
      agreement may not be approved by the Board unless the BPQA re-
      views and approves the physician's role with regard to delegated
      medical functions;
   3. Formulate standardized criteria to be used by the nurse-midwife and
      physician in developing protocols;
   4. Be available to the Board or the BPQA, or both, to review protocols
      when requested and perform any duties delegated to it by the Board
      and the BPQA.
B. The Joint Committee shall be composed of any equal number of members appointed by the Board and the BPQA. A member shall be ap-

pointed for a 3-year term and may be reappointed for one additional 3-year term.
C. Members of the Joint Committee may be members of the Board or the BPQA or may be designees of each appointing Board. The members appointed by the Board shall be certified nurse-midwives.

Nurse-Midwife Peer Review Advisory Committee

The Board shall appoint at least four certified nurse-midwives from names submitted for consideration to act as its Advisory Committee, with such powers and duties as the Board may prescribe.

Renewal of Certification

Certification as a nurse-midwife expires at the same time as the nurse-midwife's registered nursing license unless the certification is renewed.

Before a nurse-midwife's certification expires, the midwife may renew annually if the nurse-midwife:

1. Is otherwise entitled to be certified;
2. Pay to the Board all appropriate renewal fees set by the Board; and
3. Submits to the Board:
   a. A renewal application on the form that the Board requires, and
   b. Proof of enrollment in the Continuing Competency Assessment Program of the ACNM.

Unlawful Practices

Pursuant to the Health Occupations Article, Section 8-602 and 8-710, Annotated Code of Maryland, an individual may not:

A. Practice nurse-midwifery unless certified under these regulations or otherwise permitted by law to engage in those activities;
B. Use the title nurse-midwife, certified nurse-midwife, or any other similar designation unless certified by the American College of Nurse-Midwives;
C. Use the title certified nurse-midwife unless certified by the Board.

Prescribing of Substances by a Certified Nurse-Midwife

A. Pursuant to Health Occupations Article, Section 8-601, Annotated Code of Maryland, a certified nurse-midwife may:

1. Prescribe substances included in the formulary developed by the Board in consultation with the BPQA and the Pharmacy Board;
2. Prescribe controlled substances on Schedules II—V under Article 27, Section 279(b)—(e), Annotated Code of Maryland, as determined by the Board in consultation with the BPQA and the Pharmacy Board; and
3. Dispense substances prescribed in accordance with Section A(1) and (2) of this regulation in the course of treating a patient at a:
   a. Nonprofit medical facility or clinic;
   b. Health center operating on the campus of an institution of higher learning;
   c. Public health facility;
   d. Medical facility under contract with a State or local health department, or
   e. Facility funded with public funds.
B. The Board shall:
   1. Consult annually with the BPQA and the Pharmacy Board to review the formulary and make revisions as necessary; and
   2. Maintain a list of all certified nurse-midwives who are authorized to prescribe, and a record of the approved formulary which shall be made available to Maryland pharmacies through annual mailings and upon request.

BIBLIOGRAPHY

Maryland State Board of Nursing. Nurse Practice Act, Annotated Code of Maryland Health Occupations Article, Title 8, and Code of Maryland Regulations, Title 10, Subtitle 27. Baltimore: Maryland State Board of Nursing, 1995. Used by permission.

Dorsey, D, Executive Director, Maryland State Board of Nursing. (September 1995, personal communication).

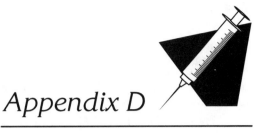

Appendix D

Code of Ethics of the American Association of Nurse Anesthetists

Preamble

The purpose of a Code of Ethics is to acknowledge a profession's acceptance of the responsibility and trust conferred upon it by society and to recognize the obligations inherent in this code. The Code of Ethics applies to nurse anesthetists who are certified (and recertified) by the Councils on Certification/Recertification of Nurse Anesthetists and AANA professionals. Certified Registered Nurse Anesthetists (CRNAs) must strive, both on an individual and collective basis, to pursue the highest possible ethical standards in rendering their services.

The principles set forth define the profession's responsibilities and expectations which each member of the AANA has a personal obligation to uphold and adhere to, as well as to ensure collegial conformance.

I. Patient Care

A Certified Registered Nurse Anesthetist has the responsibility to preserve human dignity, respect patients' rights to self-determination, and support the well-being of patients under his/her care.

Interpretation: The CRNA must render quality anesthesia care regardless of the patient's race, color, religion, age, sex, nationality, disability, or his or her social or economic status.

II. Competence

A Certified Registered Nurse Anesthetist demonstrates a high level of competence. Competence is a composite of the individual's professional values, knowledge, judgment, and technical and interpersonal skills.

Interpretation: CRNAs must assume the responsibility to strive for excellence and to maintain that level of knowledge, judgment, technical skill, and professional values prerequisite to delivering high-quality health services. CRNAs engage in lifelong professional educational activities and participate in peer review and other continuous quality-improvement mechanisms as a basis for assessing quality of care and practice, in order to ensure the public's protection. While there are no mechanisms which can fully guarantee competent practice in every instance, each CRNA joins the profession in constantly reviewing and practicing with nationally recognized standards for the public's benefit.

III. Professionalism

A Certified Registered Nurse Anesthetist is responsible and accountable for individual professional judgments and actions. The CRNA should actively support the educational process of nurse anesthetists, other health care professionals, and the public. The CRNA shall be an advocate for patients' rights and safety.

Interpretation:
A. Responsibility—A CRNA is responsible for the anesthesia care provided.
B. Professional Judgment—A CRNA is accountable for judgments made and actions taken in the practice of nurse anesthesia. Neither physicians' orders nor institutional policies relieve the CRNA of accountability for actions taken and judgments made relative to the care and well-being of patients.
C. Informed Consent—As a licensed professional, the CRNA shall verify that a valid informed consent has been obtained from the patient or legal guardian as prescribed by federal or state laws or institutional policy.
D. Safety—A CRNA shall provide quality anesthesia care and protect patients from harm.

IV. Societal Obligation

A Certified Registered Nurse Anesthetist has an obligation to society.

Interpretation: The CRNA must be a responsible citizen to society and to the community. A CRNA is obligated to be aware of environmental and global health issues.

V. Confidentiality

A Certified Registered Nurse Anesthetist protects patients' right to privacy.

Interpretation: A CRNA must maintain confidentiality of patient information unless required by law to breach the confidence.

VI. Personal Integrity

A Certified Registered Nurse Anesthetist maintains personal integrity, and strives to establish appropriate mechanisms to protect his/her freedom of conscience as it pertains to patients and to each member of the health care team.

Interpretation: A CRNA is obligated to be knowledgeable of all moral and legal rights, including those of the patient, self, and other professionals. In situations where the CRNA's personal convictions prohibit participation in a particular procedure, the CRNA may withdraw from the case, provided that such withdrawal does not harm the patient or constitute breach of duty. CRNAs should avoid employment situations where frequent conflicts of personal conviction occur.

VII. Endorsement

A Certified Registered Nurse Anesthetist may endorse products and services, provided that he/she assumes accountability for the product's safety and/or quality. A CRNA shall not act as an agent of the AANA unless duly authorized by the Board of Directors.

Interpretation: CRNAs may actively represent themselves in a variety of settings to include professional, personal, public, educational, media, and social. A CRNA must exercise sound judgment in matters which potentially involve conflict of interest in relation to the AANA.

VIII. Research Ethics

A Certified Registered Nurse Anesthetist protects patients and animals involved in research projects, and conducts the projects according to accepted ethical research and reporting standards established by public law and institutional procedures.

Interpretation:
A. The CRNA participates in research activities to expand practice and to enhance continuous quality improvement efforts.
B. The CRNA must adhere to bioethical standards in the practice setting.

IX. Practice Settings

A Certified Registered Nurse Anesthetist has the right to participate in a variety of practice settings, including private practice, institutional employment, and other variations of business organizations.

Interpretation:
   A. Right to Practice—The CRNA has the legal right to practice in a variety of employment settings and business relationships.
   B. Reimbursement Responsibility—When the CRNA is a private practitioner, he/she has an ethical responsibility to the consumer to ensure responsible reimbursement policies. Fees for professional anesthesia services should be consistent with reasonable and customary charges and reflect actual participation in, and/or consultation on, the procedure.

X. Employment Relations

A Certified Registered Nurse Anesthetist supports the profession in its efforts to maintain conditions of employment, practice privileges, and contractual relationships.

Interpretation:
   A. Responsibility for Conditions of Practice—The CRNA must practice in accordance with the standards established by the profession. These standards include the preanesthesia assessment, intraoperative management, and postanesthesia care.
   B. Contractual Agreements—The agreements shall be consistent with the professional standards of practice, laws, and/or regulations pertaining to nurse anesthesia practice.
   C. Ethical Business Practices—The CRNA should maintain ethical business practices in dealing with potential clients and colleagues. Dealings should be characterized by concepts of mutual regard, equity, honesty, and constructive interpersonal communication.

BIBLIOGRAPHY

American Association of Nurse Anesthetists. *Professional Standards and Responsibilities Regarding Patient Care.* Park Ridge, IL: American Association of Nurse Anesthetists, 1992. Used by permission.

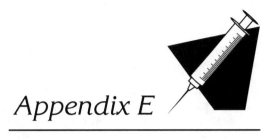

Appendix E

Practice Standards of the American Association of Nurse Anesthetists

Standard I: Perform a thorough and complete preanesthetic assessment.

Interpretation: The responsibility for the care of the patient begins with the preanesthetic assessment. Except in emergency situations, the CRNA has an obligation to complete a thorough evaluation and determine that relevant tests have been obtained and reviewed.

Standard II: Obtain informed consent for the planned anesthetic intervention from the patient or legal guardian.

Interpretation: The CRNA shall obtain or verify that an informed consent has been obtained by a qualified provider. Discuss anesthetic options and risks with the patient and/or legal guardian in language the patient and/or legal guardian can understand. Document in the patient's medical record that informed consent was obtained.

Standard III: Formulate a patient-specific plan for anesthesia care.

Interpretation: The plan of care developed by the CRNA is based upon comprehensive patient assessment, problem analysis, anticipated surgical or therapeutic procedure, patient and surgeon preferences, and current anesthesia principles.

Standard IV: Implement and adjust the anesthesia care plan based on the patient's physiological response.

Interpretation: The CRNA shall induce and maintain anesthesia at required levels. The CRNA shall continuously assess the patient's response to the anesthetic and/or surgical intervention and intervene as required to maintain the patient in a satisfactory physiologic condition.

Standard V: Monitor the patient's physiologic condition as appropriate for the type of anesthesia and specific patient needs.

Interpretation: Continuous clinical observation and vigilance are the basis of safe anesthesia care. The standard applies to all patients receiving anesthesia care and may be exceeded at any time at the discretion of the CRNA. Unless otherwise stipulated in the standards a means to monitor and evaluate the patient's status shall be immediately available for all patients. As new patient safety technologies evolve, integration into the current anesthesia practice shall be considered. The omission of any monitoring standards shall be documented and the reason stated on the patient's anesthesia record. The CRNA shall be in constant attendance of the patient until the responsibility for care has been accepted by another qualified health care provider.

A. Monitor ventilation continuously. Verify intubation of the trachea by auscultation, chest excursion, and confirmation of carbon dioxide in the expired gas. Continuously monitor end-tidal carbon dioxide during controlled or assisted ventilation. Use spirometry and ventilatory pressure monitors.

B. Monitor oxygenation continuously by clinical observation, pulse oximetry, and, if indicated, arterial blood gas analysis.

C. Monitor cardiovascular status continuously via electrocardiogram and heart sounds. Record blood pressure and heart rate at least every five minutes.

D. Monitor body temperature continuously on all pediatric patients receiving general anesthesia and, when indicated, on all other patients.

E. Monitor neuromuscular function and status when neuromuscular blocking agents are administered.

Standard VI: There shall be complete, accurate, and timely documentation of pertinent information on the patient's medical record.

Interpretation: Document all anesthetic interventions and patient responses. Accurate documentation facilitates comprehensive patient care, provides information for retrospective review and research data, and establishes a medical-legal record.

Standard VII: Transfer the responsibility for care of the patient to other qualified providers in a manner that assures continuity of care and patient safety.

Interpretation: The CRNA shall assess the patient's status and determine when it is safe to transfer the responsibility of care to other qualified providers. The CRNA shall accurately report the patient's condition and all essential information to the provider assuming responsibility for the patient.

Standard VIII: Adhere to appropriate safety precautions, as established within the institution, to minimize the risks of fire, explosion, electrical shock, and equipment malfunction. Document on the patient's medical record that the anesthesia machine and equipment were checked.

Interpretation: Prior to use, the CRNA shall inspect the anesthesia machine and monitors according to established guidelines. The CRNA shall check the readiness, availability, cleanliness, and working condition of all equipment to be utilized in the administration of the anesthesia care. When the patient is ventilated by an automatic mechanical ventilator, monitor the integrity of the breathing system with a device capable of detecting a disconnection by emitting an audible alarm. Monitor oxygen concentration continuously with an oxygen supply failure alarm system.

Standard IX: Universal precautions shall be taken to minimize the risk of infection to the patient, CRNA, and other staff.

Interpretation: Written policies and procedures in infection control shall be developed for personnel and equipment.

Standard X: Anesthesia care shall be assessed to assure its quality and contribution to positive patient outcomes.

Interpretation: The CRNA shall participate in the ongoing review and evaluation of the quality and appropriateness of anesthesia care. Evaluation shall be performed based upon appropriate outcome criteria and reviewed on an ongoing basis. The CRNA shall participate in a continual process of self-evaluation and strive to incorporate new techniques and knowledge into practice.

Standard XI: The CRNA shall respect and maintain the basic rights of patients.

Interpretation: The CRNA shall support and preserve the rights of patients to personal dignity and ethical norms of practice.

Adopted 1989
Revised 1992, 1996

BIBLIOGRAPHY

American Association of Nurse Anesthetists. *Scope and Standards for Nurse Anesthesia Practice.* Park Ridge, IL: American Association of Nurse Anesthetists, 1996. Used by permission.

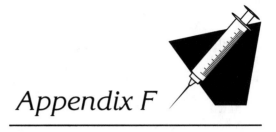

Appendix F

Maryland Nurse Practice Act and Regulations for Nurse Anesthetists

Definitions

1. "Practice of nurse anesthesia" means performing acts in collaboration with an anesthesiologist, licensed physician, or dentist which require substantial specialized knowledge, judgment, and skill related to the administration of anesthesia, including preoperative and postoperative assessment of patients; administering anesthetics; monitoring patients during anesthesia; management of fluid in intravenous therapy; respiratory care.
2. "Certified registered nurse anesthetist (CRNA)" means a registered nurse, certified by the Board and the Council of Recertification of the AANA to practice nurse anesthesia.
3. "Collaboration" means the development and implementation of an agreement between a nurse anesthetist and an anesthesiologist, licensed physician, or dentist concerning the practice of nurse anesthesia.
4. "Board" means the State Board of Nursing.
5. "AANA" means the American Association of Nurse Anesthetists.
6. "Anesthesiologist" means a Maryland licensed physician who has had special training in the field of anesthesiology, who administers anesthesia on a regular basis, and who devotes a substantial portion of his medical practice to the practice of anesthesiology.
7. "Licensed physician or dentist" as used in these regulations means one who has knowledge and experience in resuscitation, anesthetic drugs, and their reactions.

STANDARDS OF PRACTICE

1. A nurse anesthetist certified under these regulations may engage in the practice of nurse anesthesia as that term is defined in Regulation .01A above.
2. A nurse anesthetist certified under these regulations shall collaborate with an anesthesiologist, licensed physician, or dentist in the following manner:
   a. An anesthesiologist, licensed physician, or dentist shall be physically available to the nurse anesthetist for consultation at all times during the administration of and recovery from anesthesia.
   b. An anesthesiologist shall be available for consultation to the nurse anesthetist for other aspects of the practice of nurse anesthesia. If an anesthesiologist is not available, a licensed physician or dentist shall be available to provide this type of consultation.
   c. A CRNA shall report to the Board the name of the collaborating anesthesiologist, physician, or dentist. When the Board receives the name of the collaborating anesthesiologist, licensed physician, or dentist, this information shall be forwarded to the appropriate regulatory Board.
   d. A CRNA has the right and the obligation to refuse to perform any delegated act, whether oral or written, if, in the CRNA's judgment, it is an unsafe or invalidly prescribed medical act.

CERTIFICATION

An applicant for certification as a nurse anesthetist shall:

1. Hold a current license to practice registered nursing in Maryland;
2. Complete in full the application for certification as a nurse anesthetist.
3. Pay all fees established by the Board.
4. Obtain certification as a nurse anesthetist from the Council on Certification of the AANA.

A CRNA shall have this designation placed on the current license to practice as a registered nurse.

Practice Before Certification

1. A registered nurse who meets the qualifications to sit for the examinations for AANA certification and who has applied to the Council on Certification of the AANA for certification as a nurse anesthetist may

practice as a graduate nurse anesthetist (GNA) before certification in Maryland if this practice is under the supervision of an anesthesiologist.
2. A graduate nurse anesthetist may not continue to practice following denial of certification from the Council on Certification of the AANA, or for more than 2 years following the date of graduation, whichever occurs first.

Certification by Endorsement

An applicant from out-of-State applying for certification shall meet the requirements as stated in Regulation .03, above.

Renewal of Certification

To renew certification, a CRNA shall:

1. Submit a renewal application at the time the application for renewal of the license to practice registered nursing is filed;
2. Submit evidence that the recertification received from the Council on Recertification of the AANA is current, if applicable;
3. Pay all fees established by the Board.

Current Practitioners

Registered nurses who are currently practicing nurse anesthesia who do not hold certification from the Council on Certification and Council on Recertification, if applicable, of the AANA may continue to practice without Maryland certification for a period no longer than 2 years following the date of the adoption of these regulations.

CRNA ADVISORY COUNCIL

The Board shall appoint three CRNAs from a list of recommendations submitted by the Maryland Association of Nurse Anesthetists to act as its advisory council.

UNLAWFUL PRACTICES

1. Pursuant to Health Occupations Article, Title 8, Subtitle 7, Annotated Code of Maryland, a person may not:
   a. Practice nurse anesthesia unless certified under these regulations, or otherwise permitted by law to engage in these activities;
   b. Use the title nurse anesthetist, CRNA, or any other similar designation, unless certified by the Board.

2. A person certified under these regulations shall be subject to the disciplinary sanctions set forth in Health Occupations Article, Section 8-315, Annotated Code of Maryland.
3. These regulations do not limit or prohibit a registered nurse from performing those functions which constitute the practice of registered nursing as defined by law.

BIBLIOGRAPHY

Maryland State Board of Nursing. Nurse Practice Act, Annotated Code of Maryland, Health Occupations Article, Title 8, Code of Maryland Regulations, Title 10, Subtitle 27. Baltimore: Maryland Board of Nursing, 1995. Used by permission.

Appendix G

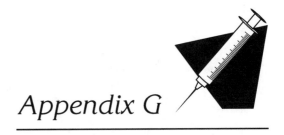

Professional Organizations of Advanced Practice Nursing

American Academy of Nurse Practitioners

Administration: Capitol Station, LBJ Building, Box 12846, Austin, TX 78711; Phone: 512-442-4262; Fax 512-442-6469.

Governmental Affairs: Box 40013, Washington, DC 20016. Publication: *Journal of the Academy of Nurse Practitioners*. Subscriptions: American Academy of Nurse Practitioners, Capitol Station, LBJ Building, Box 12846, Austin, TX 78711.

Certification Examinations for Adult and Family NPs: American Academy of Nurse Practitioners, Box 12846, Austin, TX 78711; Phone: 512-442-4262; Fax: 512-442-6469. [*Note:* Not all state boards accept certification through the Academy; inquire at the number listed.]

American Association of Colleges of Nursing

Administration: One Dupont Circle NW—Suite 530, Washington, DC 20036. Phone 202-463-6930; Fax: 202-785-8320.

American Association of Nurse Anesthetists

Administration: 222 South Prospect Avenue, Park Ridge, IL 60068-4001. Phone 708-692-7050; Fax: 708-692-6968.

Publications: *American Association of Nurse Anesthetists Journal* (bimonthly); *AANA News Bulletin* (alternate months).

American College of Nurse-Midwives

Administration: 818 Connecticut Avenue NW, Suite 900, Washington, DC 20006. Phone: 202-728-9860; Fax: 202-728-9897.

Publication: *Journal of Nurse Midwifery* (quarterly).

American College of Nurse Practitioners

Administration: 2401 Pennsylvania Avenue NW, Washington, DC 20037-1718. Phone: 202-466-4825; Fax 202-466-3825.

Publication: *The Nurse Practitioner—The American Journal of Primary Care Health Care.*

American Nurses Credentialing Center

Administration: 600 Maryland Avenue SW, Suite 100 West, Washington, DC 20024-2571. Phone (membership): 800-274-4262; Phone (application forms): 800-284-CERT.

National Association of Nurse Practitioners in Reproductive Health

Administration: 2401 Pennsylvania Avenue NW, Washington, DC 20037-1718. Phone: 202-466-4825.

National Certification Corporation for the Obstetric, Gynecologic, and Neonatal Nursing Specialties

Administration: Box 11082, Chicago, IL 60611-0082. Phone: 312-951-0207 or 800-367-5613.

National Organization of Clinical Nurse Specialists

Contact: Cathy Brown, Executive Director, National Association of Clinical Nurse Specialists, 101 Columbia, Aliso Viejo, CA 92656. Phone: 800-452-4467.

Publication: *The Journal for Advanced Practice Nursing* (bimonthly).

National Organization of Nurse Practitioner Faculties

Administration: One Dupont Circle NW, Washington, DC 20036. Phone: 202-463-6930; Fax: 202-785-8320.

Publications: *Guidelines for Nurse Practitioner Curriculums and Educational Program Standards; Directory of Nurse Practitioner Programs; Nurse Practitioner Faculty Practice Models;* and others.

Index